Wim Distelmans is an oncologist and professor of palliat
Free University of Brussels, Belgium. He has campaignec
of palliative care and striven for the (legal) right to a cho
(euthanasia). He has been awarded several prizes: the Ar
Word (2003), the Tenrei Ohta Award of the World Federation of Right to Die
Societies (2008), the Ignis Fatuus Prize (2010), the Lucien Steinberg Prize
for Medical Research (2012), the Award for Societal Valorisation of the Free
University of Brussels (2012), 'ambassador' of the Christian-oriented David
Foundation (2012) and the Liberal Humanism Prize (2015). He is, amongst
other things, president of the Forum for Palliative Care, the palliative
home team Omega and the Cédric Hèle Institute (Flemish Institute for
Psychosocial Oncology). Together with the University Hospital Brussels, he
founded Topaz, the first palliative and supportive day-care centre in Belgium,
and the interdisciplinary 'rescue' consultation group UL Team, aimed at
elucidating difficult end-of-life requests (including euthanasia). He is holder
of the Dignified Life's End chair of the Belgian Liberal Society (deMens.nu)
at the Free University of Brussels. He is founder and president of the Life's
End Information Forum (LEIF) and co-president of the Belgian Federal
Euthanasia Commission. He established these initiatives at the Dignified
Life's End expertise centre at Wemmel, close to Brussels.

The Flemish edition of this book (*Een Waardig Levenseinde*) has become a
bestseller, a ninth revised edition of which was published recently.

*As a child I always wanted to be a 'do-gooder', and Albert Schweitzer was
my absolute hero. Hence, after finishing medical school I went to the Institute
of Tropical Medicine in Antwerp and got a licence in tropical medicine. For
several years I worked for a UN project aiming to eradicate sleeping sickness
in Nigeria. For political and financial reasons the project was abandoned
in 1982. Fortunately, I got the opportunity to continue my 'humanitarian'
ambitions by doing basic research on cancer. One of the anti-cancer products
I worked on I was able personally to patent. However, I realised quite soon
that despite all therapeutic and research efforts about 50 per cent of all cancer
patients remain untreatable and eventually die. Unlike in the UK, there
existed no valuable support for these patients in Belgium. So we organised
several study trips to England and Scotland to improve our knowledge of
palliative care. Subsequently, we introduced specialised palliative care in
Belgium and for years we tried to convince the government to support it
sufficiently. In 1996, I became president of the first palliative initiative in
Belgium, the home-care team Omega, and launched various other palliative
care organisations. But after several years of experience with palliation, it
became very clear to open-minded health professionals that even with perfect
palliative care there will always remain a number of patients whose suffering
cannot be sufficiently relieved. For that reason, alongside our efforts on the
further implementation of palliative care, I strongly concentrated on the
possibility of creating a legal framework for a self-chosen death, or euthanasia.*

In the Western world there remains a stark contrast between the quality of life and the quality of death.

In Pursuit of a
Dignified Life's End

The Belgian Model

Wim Distelmans

translated by Jacqueline Balfour

Hartfield Publishing • London

Published in 2015 by Hartfield Publishing
Aston House
Cornwall Avenue
London
N3 1LF

ISBN 978-0-9932686-0-1

A full CIP record for this book is available from the British Library

Typeset in Minion by Dexter Haven Associates Ltd, London
Printed in Great Britain by TJ International, Padstow

Contents

The greatest mistake in the treatment of diseases is that there are physicians for the body and physicians for the soul, although the two cannot be separated.

Plato

Thought must never submit,
neither to a dogma, nor to a party,
nor to a passion, nor to an interest,
nor to a preconceived idea, nor to whatever it may be,
save to the facts themselves,
because, for thought, submission would mean ceasing to be.

Henri Poincaré
Philosopher of Science

Although palliative care teams should in theory render themselves redundant, they will in practice always exist. It is the only way to reduce futile persistence.

Derek Doyle
Oxford Textbook of Palliative Medicine

Life is a gift from God. Once it is over, you can give it back.

Harry Kuitert
Theologian

Concern for man himself and his fate must always form the chief interest of all technical endeavours.

Albert Einstein
Nobel Prize winner

The dying in our society are to an ever-increasing extent, neither owner nor master of their dying process.

They are largely controlled (willingly or unwillingly) by medics and paramedics and are spoken about as medical objects rather than as people.

They no longer live their last days, they experience them. Their end of life becomes 'undignified'.

The dying are forced into human self-alienation and reduced to passive 'impersonal' spectators of their own dying process, as if it was that of a stranger.

So let us not mince our words because treading softly around the issue keeps us blind to the bitter reality: it is high time we realise that desubjectification is an institutionalised social assault on man as an autonomous person.

Professor Hugo Van den Enden (1937–2007)
Philosopher and Moral Scientist, University of Ghent, Belgium

Foreword
Manu Keirse

A Dignified Life's End means different things to different people in different parts of the world. For some it is automatically associated with the 'right to die with dignity' movement, which in turn is very quickly associated with euthanasia. This book does not promote euthanasia as the only way to die with dignity. It looks at a much broader history of human illness. It casts a critical eye over the ways in which the technology available to doctors today can be used either to promote or hinder human well-being. The author's response to the question of a dignified death is not restricted to a discussion about euthanasia, but rather about the dignified use of the whole range of medical options available today.

As an oncologist, Wim Distelmans asks critical questions about the ways in which medical decisions are made. Do they always result in the patient's improved well-being, or can they sometimes be a burden rather than a benefit to the patient? He not only asks questions but also clearly illustrates how the failure adequately to weigh up which medical techniques to use – based on the given patient, the circumstances, the time period and the purpose of the treatment – can burden the patient more than help them. This book is not primarily about medical technology, but about how it is used and its appropriateness.

This book, from beginning to end, is also a plea for patients to be considered as whole people with their own feelings and their own understanding of the situation, their own norms and values and perception of quality of life. It focuses not only on the dying process, as some may assume from its title, but also on the process of living with a life-threatening illness. The author maintains that medical interventions can guarantee maximum comfort, provided they are adequately administered in the right context. This book is peppered with inspiring suggestions. When evaluating the use of radiotherapy or chemotherapy to treat a tumour it is important to consider not only whether the tumour has reduced in size, but also to find out how the patient is responding to the treatment; does it induce vomiting? Has the patient lost weight? Are they suffering in other ways? The author bases his choices of treatment not only on what scientific and medical opinion would consider to be the best possible choice, but also considers each option within the context of each individual patient, as a whole. This seems obvious, but those who are familiar with the practice know that it is not always easy, and requires good communication skills. This is referred to in the new Belgian Law on Patients' Rights, which expressly stipulates that each patient must give their consent for all research and all treatment, after they have been fully informed about any possible side-effects and consequences.

Throughout the entire book, he also illustrates that qualitative medicine is based on open informed communication with the patient. It is only possible to talk about patient autonomy and patient participation if the patient is fully and reliably informed of all possible eventualities, the expected benefits and the side-effects of the treatments. The author believes that this can only work in a multidisciplinary group, including psycho-social and ideological experts as full partners of the team providing input.

The title – *In Pursuit of a Dignified Life's End* – therefore also describes a book that demonstrates how medicine can be degrading if not appropriate for the patient's needs, values, beliefs and perception of the situation. The many insights in this book show that we can enjoy life thanks to the responsible use of the medical options.

Medical professionals pledge to prioritise comfort and quality of life during treatment, even if this is compromised by the life-threatening nature of the disease. The book draws on palliative care and palliative medicine and opens windows that give a view of humanity in the healthcare sector. The author also refers to pioneers in palliative care and treatment, such as Dame Cicely Saunders, who founded the first hospice for terminally ill people, St Christopher's, in London. She is widely recognised as the founder of the palliative-care movement. It is perhaps symbolic that I first considered the work the author has conducted on these issues while Dame Cicely Saunders herself was dying in the hospice that she founded in 1967. It must have been very satisfying for her, someone who truly broke ground, to see her torch being carried forward by others.

This book will undoubtedly cause many people to rethink their views on how modern medicine can best be used for the service of humankind. For this reason it is desirable that it should be read not only by doctors working in palliative care, but also by all specialists and general practitioners, nurses and other healthcare providers who come into contact with life-threatening illnesses.

It is also a book that offers patients and family members more opportunities to defend themselves in such situations. Playing an active role in one's treatment requires sufficient knowledge and information. The author also regularly refers to the Patients' Rights Law, which recognises the right to information and to active participation as a central element of human dignity. The stress of living with a serious illness is often as much of a burden for loved ones as for the patient, and everyone should inform themselves about these issues before being confronted with them in reality. Uninformed participation always leads to empty opinions. It is better to consider the options available and what we would like for the end of our own lives in advance. Dying is always living 'the last moments of life' and who wouldn't prefer to determine this for themselves?

Manu Keirse is Professor Emeritus at the Faculty of Medicine of the Catholic University of Leuven, and President of the Belgian Federal Palliative Care Assessment Unit

Preface

This book was inspired by my huge aversion for any form of patronisation. In my daily dealings with serious, incurable illness, I am repeatedly struck by how much we as healthcare professionals tend to want to decide everything for the patient and their families, and how little respect and patience we show them.

This book aims to provide (future) patients and their families with sufficient information to be able to make informed decisions for themselves. It is also aimed at healthcare professionals who want to treat the seriously ill with respect and empathy, not only during the dying process, but throughout the illness.

In 2002 the three laws relating to end of life – unique to Belgium – were voted into law: the Patients' Rights Law, the Palliative Care Law and the Euthanasia Law. This book attempts to give an overview of the origins of care and end-of-life decisions, and how they have evolved in Belgium.

I hope this book will contribute to the public debate in countries where these basic human and patients' rights are not yet available.

If just one seriously ill patient is spared unnecessary suffering as a result of this book, then I will consider it to have been a success.

Introduction

In the mid-eighties, a group of carers in various parts of Flanders, the Dutch-speaking part of Belgium, took the first tentative initiatives to provide terminally ill patients in their dying days with better support. The first 'palliative' home-care teams were born, consisting, in reality, almost exclusively of volunteers. Often only a few technical devices, such as syringe drivers to administer regular pain relief, were provided for, thanks to local service clubs or 'people's fairs'. These pioneers were made of stern stuff and learnt their craft by trial and error.

Instigated by Lisette Custermans – a psychiatric nurse from the Faculty of Medicine at the Vrije Universiteit Brussel and founder of the first fully fledged palliative care provision in Belgium, Palliative Home Care Omega – these *avant la lettre* palliative experts met regularly. The main topic of discussion at these meetings was how difficult it is to convince regular healthcare professionals of the importance of good end-of-life care. Occasionally there would be small-scale training with a speaker from England, where the palliative care movement started, and where interestingly there is now an intense debate on the subject of euthanasia.

In 1990 Sister Leontine founded the first hospice in the St John's Hospital in Brussels with the support of the royal family. At around the same time, palliative care teams were formed in a few large hospitals.

I started working on the development of palliative care from the beginning. As an oncologist, I witness daily how seriously ill or incurable cancer patients require proper support. We organised training throughout

Flanders, in backrooms in cafés, in bare parish halls, in big and small cultural centres. There was huge demand from healthcare professionals who were caring for seriously ill patients, daily, patients who were being given all kinds of futile treatment with very little concern for the pain that might result, or the psychological impact.

Erik Vanden Abeele, from the pharmaceutical company in Puurs, Upjohn (as it then was; it is now, after several painful mergers, part of Pfizer) put me in touch with his colleague and project leader Tony De Bondt. Together, in 1994, we organised the first large-scale Palliative Care Conference in Flanders in a conference centre in Baarle. It was an immediate success and we were forced to turn people away due to lack of space.

Palliative care had arrived in Flanders to stay. Since then there has been a steady stream of lectures, symposia and training, as well as very well attended study trips to England, Scotland, Russia and more recently Poland with Thierry Van Calster. The only thing missing was money. Due to an unforeseen consensus between people from all different walks of life and ideologies, several ministerial cabinets were spliced together to get the much-needed resources. At the beginning and indeed today, Flemish palliative care survives and grows due to the continued and prominent support from Vic Anciaux, Leo Leys and Kathy Lindekens of the national action group Kom op tegen Kanker.

At the beginning of 1990, thanks to pressure from Philippe Busquin, the former Federal Minister of Social Affairs, the first moves towards state funding were made. It took ten years of pressure before a reasonable fund was provided. During this inefficient progression, the compassionate attitude of Dr Georges Vereecke, from the Belgian National Institute for Health and Disability Insurance, was highly appreciated.

There followed the first real recognition of the need for distinct palliative care provision from the Government: from former federal ministers Magda Aelvoet (public health) and Frank Vandenbroucke (social affairs), as well as other interested parties such as Chris Decoster, Manu Keirse, Paul Verhaevert and Rik Thys.

In addition to the rise, in recent years, of palliative care there has been a concurrent campaign for the right for greater choice over when we die, or euthanasia. In 1983, Leon Favyts, founder of the Flemish Right to Die

Society (RWS) and Hugo Van den Enden, Professor of Philosophy and Moral Science at the University of Ghent, recruited many in favour of legislation on euthanasia to their association.

Although, despite support from many, a significant number of palliative care initiatives failed initially for ideological or other reasons, there were also many who supported the possibility of euthanasia from the beginning.

Much to the astonishment of both its opponents and proponents, the Euthanasia Bill proposed by Senators Jeannine Leduc, Myriam Vanlerberghe, Jacinta De Roeck, Philippe Mahoux, Philippe Monfils and Marie Nagy was voted into Belgian law by the purple–green (Socialists–Liberals–Greens) majority.

Euthanasia, however, is just one of an infinite number of end-of-life decisions. Figures from research into the end of life performed under Luc Deliens illustrate all too clearly the influence that doctors have on the ends of our lives.

Both civilians and professionals need clear impartial information about the end of life, which is why a Life's End Information Forum (Levens Einde Informatie Forum, LEIF) was set up with specialised doctors and the telephone helpline LEIF line. From the beginning this forum was manned by me and Paul Destrooper, along with an increasing number of highly committed people: Christine Van Broeckhoven, Rik Torfs, Sabien Bauwens, Patrik Vankrunkelsven, Joke Denekens, Etienne De Groot, Raymond Mathys, Jef Vermassen, Magrit De Maegd, Reinier Hueting, Colette Raymakers, Johan Bilsen, Kris Van de Gaer, Celesta Saerens, Katrien Van Rossum and Sven Claessens. It also received immediate support from the former Flemish minister Adelheid Byttebier. The concept of the welcoming 'house style' was the brainwave of Jean-Luc Servais (a French-speaking Fleming or bilingual Belgian with roots in Brussels-Halle-Vilvoorde), the result of his sympathy and commitment to the project. Later, despite troubled times in the state budget, LEIF received a symbolic boost from Rudy Demotte.

The global public debate about death and dying is very closely followed by the fourth power in our country: the media. Top journalists such as Yves Desmet from *De Morgen*, Guy Tegenbos from *De Standaard* and Jan

Lippens from the weekly *Humo* have given tireless support to the debate with frequent well-aimed metaphorical punches from their corners.

I have never understood how it is possible, in a pluralistic, multicultural society, on the one hand to talk about 'respect for the patient' and on the other to give all the possible options for a dignified end of life different weight. Experience clearly shows that many patients are very grateful for palliative care, *if they are offered it*. Others choose, immediately or some time during their treatment, a self-determined death – *provided* their request is heard and honoured.

Compared to our neighbours – except for the Netherlands and recently Luxembourg – we can consider ourselves lucky. On a global scale Belgium is also a notable exception. Of course there is still room for improvement, but Belgium is the only country in the world to have a Palliative Care Law and a Euthanasia Law. In Switzerland and some states in the USA – Oregon, Washington, Montana and Vermont – only self-administered assisted dying is available. The terminally ill patient is given the drugs or prescription and they must administer them themselves.

Fortunately the earlier, often heated and emotional, debate about the Euthanasia Law has subsided among palliative care teams who are most often confronted by it, but debate about end-of-life care has now gained momentum among other healthcare providers. Only fundamentalists, pressure groups and sensation-seeking (foreign) media continue to show little or no respect for the final wishes of those in unbearable suffering.

It remains a privilege to be able to participate in one of the most interesting bio-ethical developments of the last few decades. This book will provide greater insight into end-of-life care. It is written for anyone who wants to be empowered in a medicalised world. It is also specifically aimed at healthcare professionals who want to treat their patients with empathy.

The book is based on years of training and lectures on palliative care and end-of-life decisions including euthanasia, not least with my dear friend Etienne de Groot.

I hope above all that this book modestly contributes to the urgently needed change in attitude towards all incurable patients to ensure respect for their individuality and to avoid therapeutic obstinacy.

The book begins with a description of past highlights. It then looks at the main problems and ethical questions with which we are confronted in practice. Technical information is kept to a minimum and the book is written, as far as possible, in layman's terms. Only the main principles of usable medications are given. In Anglo-Saxon literature there exist numerous excellent books about chronic pain medication and other palliative tools.

My writing style may, at times, come across as being very militant and lacking in nuance. One reason for this is my desire, within a limited context, to get my views on an undignified end of life across.

In addition, the book was written by a doctor and this will undoubtedly have affected its objectivity. All my observations about the behaviour of doctors may also apply to me.

Finally, I very much hope to be able to show that for a patient in Belgium any alleged polarisation between palliative care and euthanasia is of no importance and only still exists in the spirit of some opinion-formers.

Wim Distelmans
La Turbie, Eze, La Faurie and Brussels
Spring 2015

1 Dying without unnecessary suffering

I am not afraid of dying,
I am afraid of a painful death

Ovidius

Euthanasia, or actively choosing to end one's life with the help of a doctor, is not commonplace. In Belgium it is estimated that registered euthanasia accounts for approximately 2 per cent of all deaths each year. With around a hundred thousand deaths annually this means two thousand people per year, or six people out of three hundred dying each day do so by euthanasia, yet it remains a source of much controversy.

Aside from euthanasia, there are five other decisions that can be taken to affect our dying process. These include:

- stopping or not commencing with a (futile) treatment;
- an increase in pain relief which results in death, but death is not the intention (the doctrine of double effect);
- palliative sedation;
- unrequested life termination (sometimes called 'non-voluntary' euthanasia in Anglo-Saxon countries: see p. 11);
- assisted suicide or assisted dying.

These options are chosen 25 times more frequently than euthanasia – sometimes without the patient knowing about it – but are often conflated.

Few people have a clear understanding of these choices and how they differ; therefore they are discussed in detail in this book.

Why is there still such resistance to euthanasia?

'Euthanatos' in ancient Greek means 'good, easy death' but over time it has frequently been given a different meaning. The worst abuse of this concept was in Nazi Germany, when the Nazis spoke of the T4 'Euthanasieprogramm' when they started systematically to kill all those they considered to be inferior: those with mental disabilities or psychiatric problems, and later homosexuals, Gypsies and Jews. Opponents of the possibilities offered by euthanasia often base their arguments on these practices.

In addition, many opponents inspired by Christianity state the translation of the famous Hebrew quote from the Bible 'lo tirtsah', which they incorrectly translate as 'Thou shalt not kill', although it would be more correctly translated as 'Thou shalt not murder'.

Fortunately the Belgian Advisory Committee on Bioethics took the initiative in 1997 to provide a clear definition of euthanasia and thus eliminate other erroneous definitions. Since then in Belgium euthanasia is taken to mean 'the intentional termination of the life (by a doctor) of a patient who has expressly requested it and which complies with certain prerequisite conditions'.

Nevertheless, the term euthanasia is still frequently used incorrectly. One often hears people saying they are going to 'euthanise' their dogs, or that they would like to commit 'euthanasia' on their interfering mother-in-law. Since neither of the above have expressly asked for it they cannot be euthanised. A person can put a dog to sleep or give it a lethal injection or, expressed more technically, terminate its life without being asked to by the dog. One doesn't usually talk about committing euthanasia, but rather performing or carrying out euthanasia. One commits murder and performs euthanasia.

The definition of the term 'euthanasia' is less strictly applied in countries where euthanasia is not legislated for, such as the UK, the USA and Canada, and continues to create confusion. In these countries it is widely believed that euthanasia is the intentional termination of life at the request of the patient, but also sometimes *without* the patient requesting it. This explains why these countries responded so emotionally when the Belgian Euthanasia Law was extended to include minors *with 'the capacity of discernment'*. It was wrongly assumed that all minors in Belgium could now be 'euthanised' without specifically requesting it.

Further on in this book, I try to explain why many doctors, in Belgium and elsewhere, still have so much trouble with euthanasia.

Why does euthanasia play so much on people's imaginations?

If you discuss euthanasia with a journalist, you can be sure there'll be an article about it in the media. If you discuss palliative or terminal care, the journalist doesn't even listen to what you have to say. It seems that euthanasia is a 'media-friendly' issue that plays on our imaginations.

Euthanasia results in death but the patient specifically requests it. The feeling of liberation introduced by the Euthanasia Law in Belgium should not be underestimated. Thanks to this law more and more people are realising that they can be proactive in their own death. More and more doctors hear their patients saying that they want 'their papers to be in order'. People no longer want to approach death with their eyes closed, but want to record their wishes in advance.

This is the groundbreaking impact of the current Euthanasia Law. Belgians don't want to lose the right to control the end of their lives – not only through euthanasia – and in fact want to extend this right to the whole diagnostic process. As soon as a serious illness has been diagnosed, they want to be involved in every decision. They no longer accept that medical decisions – not only questions of life and death – should be taken unilaterally by the doctors. They want to be informed as much as possible and have a say in the decisions.

Later there will be an explanation of the various choices at the end of life in our current high-tech society. I hope that after reading it the reader will be sufficiently well informed to play a more active role – if they would like to – in determining the circumstances of their own death. In this way much unnecessary suffering can be avoided.

End of life in today's technological world

In our high-tech world, people are no longer concerned with life and death. The world is full of many fantastic and abundant possibilities – cars, aeroplanes, the internet, iPads, gastronomy, movies and books: the sky is the limit. All of these developments have been universally available in Western Europe for a mere fifty years. Developments in the medical field are equally staggering. The development of medical technology really took off in the sixties and is still on the increase. It was a time of great euphoria because humans had made significant strides in combating illness, pain and death. Today, it is hard to imagine how people must have suffered over the last million years: effective painkillers such as morphine have only been available for around a hundred years. Modern high-tech medical technology alleviates much suffering: people are living longer and their quality of life has improved thanks to certain treatments and interventions. We are the first generation to be able to influence both the beginning and the end of life. Think of in-vitro fertilisation and the feeding tube.

But now, with fifty years' experience of cutting-edge medical technology, we realise more and more that this new technology can also be responsible for increased suffering. This occurs when therapeutic options are used inappropriately or for too long. In fact this so-called 'therapeutic persistence' rather than 'prolonging life' creates a 'prolonged dying process'.

It is no coincidence that, with fifty years' experience of the advantages and disadvantages of medical technology and the ageing population, a debate has been sparked in many countries about decisions that affect peoples' deaths, futile medical treatment and the alternative: palliative care. People are now beginning to question whether keeping someone alive artificially using all the available technology such as feeding tubes and artificial respiration is always the best option. These questions were not necessary fifty years ago, since these life-prolonging techniques were not then available. People died in sometimes appalling conditions and only if they were lucky or had money, in the presence of a priest and a doctor. But in fact neither of these two could do much more than other bystanders except monitor the patient until they were dead while trying to comfort them with claims that their suffering was for a reason and of a better 'afterlife'.

With the availability of life-prolonging technology, ethical thinking about death has taken on a new dimension.

Medically influenced end of life

In the past we all used to die 'natural' deaths. We would die as a result of an illness, infection or accident. Today things have changed. In at least half of all deaths, the time of death is determined by a prior decision. There are six decisions that can or should be taken because patients and their doctors have become dependent on the available medical technology. As previously mentioned these decisions are: stopping or not commencing with a (futile) treatment, an increase in pain relief which results in death, but where death is not the intention (the doctrine of double effect), palliative sedation, unrequested life termination (sometimes wrongly called non-voluntary euthanasia), assisted suicide or dying and euthanasia. Yet, despite all medical possibilities in our modern, hectic society, we will all at some point be confronted with someone dying a painful death. (We've all heard statements and questions like 'Is it normal that Dad is in so much pain?', 'I can't take it anymore, please put an end to it', 'I can't talk to my wife about my situation', 'The doctors say there is nothing more that they can do for my mother', 'I don't want my child to suffer any more'.) Dying is bad enough in itself but it becomes unbearable when accompanied by *avoidable* pain and suffering.

In the West about one in a hundred people die annually. In Belgium, around three hundred people die every day; in the UK it is more in the region of one thousand eight hundred. It is understandable, therefore, that the subject of death is difficult for most people. An undignified death is not only hard for the patient and their family, but also makes the grieving process very difficult. In addition, it often leads to skyrocketing health costs, absenteeism at work, 'doctor shopping' and resorting to questionable alternative medicine.

One possible explanation would be the explosion in medical technology during the last half century, which as previously mentioned can reduce or eliminate pain but can equally lead to increased suffering.

Biomedical research has indeed provided many sophisticated diagnostic and therapeutic options, often to the extent that more attention is given to the technology than to the needs of the patient.

The advent of the internet and multimedia has meant that people are more empowered, while at the same time healthcare professionals are realising increasingly that medical technology will never be able to solve all health problems. The possibilities of medical technology are not infinite.

As a result, reactive movements formed in most industrialised countries. On the one hand were those who advocated the right to choose one's own death (or euthanasia) and on the other were those who felt that terminally ill people should be treated with empathy and given professional palliative care, the main concern of this latter group being quality of life for terminally ill people followed by a dignified death free of any futile therapeutic persistence. In a broader sense, both groups recognised a need to promote a change in attitude among healthcare professionals and society in general. The ultimate goal should always be the humane treatment of the incurably ill. This vision not only needs to be seamlessly integrated into the care system, but also requires changes to the training given to healthcare providers.

Medical training (especially for doctors) places too much emphasis on the use of technology for acute and/or curable diseases. Doctors are still trained to be paternalistic and expect limited input from the patient. A surgeon confronted with a case of acute appendicitis will inform the patient that they need an urgent operation. The doctor knows that this is the best course of action in this situation so chooses not to consult with the patient but makes a unilateral, paternalistic decision.

Healthcare is not, however, only about acute illnesses but also includes numerous chronic, incurable diseases which will only increase with the ageing population.

Life is a disease; and the only difference between one man and another is the stage of the disease at which he lives. (George Bernard Shaw)

When dealing with terminally ill patients, doctors – in addition to giving life-prolonging treatment – can only try to improve the quality of their remaining time. Providing the maximum living and dying comfort is only possible in consultation with the patient; once informed of their medical condition in terms that they understand, the patient knows better than anyone what they perceive as *their* acceptable quality of life and quality of dying. The doctor is the medical expert but the patient is the 'human' expert on themselves. The best result will come from dialogue between the two.

The doctor's paternalistic attitude – positive when dealing with acute illnesses – is also applied daily in situations where it becomes negative. A doctor's training conditions them to take unilateral decisions about further treatment. When dealing with chronic suffering, doctors are inclined to treat them in much the same way as acute problems, constantly considering different therapeutic options. Doctors are trained to have an aversion to therapeutic checkmate. If one therapy fails, they move on to the next without stopping to consider whether it is a sensible solution.

As a result, existing technology is used inappropriately, thus failing in its purpose, which is to promote the quality of life of incurable patients. There is no point in using cutting-edge technology just because it is available. An elderly man in a care home may prefer not to visit the hospital regularly during his last weeks for brain metastasis radiotherapy but rather to have his grandchildren visit him in a familiar room despite the physical discomfort. We can only know this by reading his thoughts, or by asking him.

The patient sets the scene, the healthcare professionals do their best to make it happen

Care providers therefore need to adjust their thinking and accept *again* that there are still incurable diseases and that life is finite.

They also need to undergo thorough training in communication skills, pain and symptom control as well as psychological and spiritual support. Very little attention is paid to death despite it being the most common disorder of all. It can be summed up as follows: medical faculties continue stubbornly to maintain that chronic diseases can only be eradicated by ploughing all resources into the development of medical technology, thereby overlooking whole-patient care and symptom control. The basic curriculum of future doctors should therefore be reviewed as a matter of urgency in all universities.

Palliative care and self-chosen death

Palliative care covers all incurable ailments and can easily be administered in conjunction with the phasing out of (what has become) futile medical treatment. The two are not mutually exclusive. Psychosocial care or pain control must also be possible during chemotherapy treatment, for example.

For many this means acceptable levels of comfort during their final days. For others, the quality of life is not acceptable. Fortunately, in Belgium, it has been possible for over ten years to choose to die (euthanasia) in certain circumstances. Here again palliative care and euthanasia are not mutually exclusive. After being given detailed information about palliative care options, some people may opt directly for euthanasia whereas others may only start considering euthanasia during palliative care.

What does the term 'palliative care' mean?

To Cure Sometimes,
Relieve Often
and Care Always
(*Ambroise Paré*)

The term 'palliation' or 'palliative' comes from the Latin verb 'palliare' which means 'to cover with a cloak' (pallium) or 'to cover up' and, derived from this, 'to hold', 'to hide' or 'to soften'. Palliative care entails doing everything possible to neutralise or at least reduce the complications and symptoms caused by an incurable condition. Palliative care was originally intended, (particularly in the UK) for incurable cancer patients. And today still, 80 per cent of palliative care patients are cancer sufferers.

Palliative care is universally applicable and globally important. Worldwide more than a million people die each week. Of these, about 60 per cent would benefit from some form of palliative care.

The most used and recent definition of palliative care by the World Health Organisation in Geneva (2002) is the following:

> Palliative care is an approach that improves the quality of life of patients and their families facing the problem associated with life-threatening illness, through the prevention and relief of suffering by means of early identification and impeccable assessment and treatment of pain and other problems, physical, psychosocial and spiritual.
>
> Palliative care:
> - provides relief from pain and other distressing symptoms;
> - affirms life and regards dying as a normal process;
> - intends neither to hasten or postpone death;
> - integrates the psychological and spiritual aspects of patient care;
> - offers a support system to help patients live as actively as possible until death;
> - offers a support system to help the family cope during the patient's illness and in their own bereavement;
> - uses a team approach to address the needs of patients and their families, including bereavement counselling, if indicated;
> - will enhance quality of life, and may also positively influence the course of illness;
> - is applicable early in the course of illness, in conjunction with other therapies that are intended to prolong life, such as chemotherapy or radiation therapy, and includes those investigations needed to better understand and manage distressing clinical complications.

Quite a mouthful, but as a definition it is important because it forms the perfect basis from which to derive the basic concepts of palliative care and its evolution.

Palliative care versus palliative medicine

The original intention behind palliative *care* (also called terminal care) was the support for patients with weeks, or at best months, left to live. Palliative *medicine*, as opposed to curative medicine, is about palliation versus curing. It is the treatment of incurable, but not (as yet) terminal conditions. Palliative care can be seen as a possible end phase to palliative medicine, when the complications are so severe that they require specialised care.

Another way to describe it is as follows. Both curative medicine and palliative medicine are *active* treatments of the disease itself, which can still be controlled or affected. An example of active treatment is the cessation, or at least the slowing down, of the spread of cancer. Active treatment is curative if the disease can be controlled in such a way that it is fully cured (curative medicine or curative therapy). Active treatment is palliative if the disease is affected, possibly prolonging life, but not cured (palliative medicine or palliative therapy). Active therapy in both instances – with a palliative or curative intention – makes use of the latest technology. In the treatment of cancer this is surgery, radiotherapy and chemotherapy.

Palliative care, on the other hand, aims to alleviate the discomfort of an incurable disease rather that to fight the disease itself. An incurable disease in chronic or terminal patients also has a clear impact on the patients' emotions, family and social network. For this reason, much attention is also paid to the psychological, spiritual and family context.

Curative medicine	}	'active treatment'
Palliative medicine		use of latest technology
		not yet terminal
Palliative terminal care		limited use of the latest technology
		weeks, months to live

It becomes more complicated when the term 'palliative care' is used as a general description. People think of palliative care more as an attitude or movement within healthcare services where the incurable patient and their family play a central role. The movement started in England and was known as the hospice movement (because it started in the established hospices (see below). It later came to be known as the palliative movement.

The palliative care movement as a social movement puts the focus on the terminally ill patient and their family. The patient calls the shots and the care providers do their best to follow.

Palliative care is multidimensional

The merit of palliative care is that it focuses not only on the disease but also on the patient and their family and those who care for them. In curative medicine, the patient is considered more as an entity with a defective part needing repair (disease-oriented approach), whereas in the palliative phase the focus is also on the impact of the defective part (the incurable problem) on the patient and their family (patient-oriented approach).

The term 'total pain'

Any given complaint – physical (pain, vomiting) or mental (confusion and fear) – is affected by other influences. The concept of 'total pain' was first introduced by Dame Cicely Saunders, the pioneer of palliative care in the UK, decades ago.

It can be described as follows. Pain stimuli in the nerve endings send impulses via the nervous system to the cerebral cortex. These then translate into pain sensations and are experienced as pain. In the cerebral cortex, however, there are many other factors that influence the pain sensation and can alter it considerably. Pain caused by a new bone metastasis will have a totally different meaning for the person concerned than pain caused by a sports trauma in a gym. The fear of death makes the bone pain in the first instance more difficult to control. The impact of other key factors – such as depression, insomnia, irritability, emotional problems, difficulties with the children, a painful divorce, social problems, financial difficulties and spiritual distress, for example – should not be underestimated. Even a partial solution to these problems is enough to allow the level of painkillers to be kept constant for long periods of time.

On the other hand, there are patients whose past makes it virtually impossible to eliminate or make the pain bearable despite all the available tools. Consider, for example, a woman with an incestuous history. A painful uterine cancer can rake up unpleasant memories of her past.

All symptoms must be considered in the broader context. One could therefore also talk about 'total vomiting' and 'total confusion'.

Being sick is multidimensional

A serious illness means more than physical and psychological symptoms. One often speaks of the four dimensions:

- pain and symptoms;
- psychological problems;
- social welfare;
- spiritual and existential needs.

In addition to the physical and psychological symptoms, a serious disease can have a negative psychological impact on the patient and their family, resulting in financial difficulties, perhaps, or giving rise to other existential questions. All these dimensions interact with each other, and so it is important to help the patient and their family to have the best quality of life possible.

Palliative care involves more than holding hands and caressing the patient in soft candlelight. It is a professional approach to the complexity of serious illness. Even sitting quietly with the patient – active listening – and remaining attentive to any verbal or non-verbal communication from the patient can help. This is only possible with good training and a thorough knowledge of the patient's file.

Healthcare professionals are not superheroes. They cannot be experts in all of the four dimensions, and therefore have to work in teams. The patient and their family (not the doctor) must be the central focus, and all decisions must be taken with them and their wellbeing in mind. Consultations between various disciplines are known as interdisciplinary collaboration, which is not the same as a multidisciplinary work, where several specialists consult in a medical centre, but without obligatory contact or cooperation.

Palliative care places a strong emphasis on interdisciplinary work, a form of collaboration which should be practised in all branches of healthcare.

The structure for these consultations is horizontal rather than hierarchical. Everyone's contribution, although not equal, is of equal value because each one has specific expertise in a different aspect of the care. The importance of the role of each team member will vary as the disease evolves. If paying the hospital bill creates financial concerns for the family, the role of the social worker is very important, whereas if the pain is the predominant

FIGURE 1   INTERDISCIPLINARY WORK

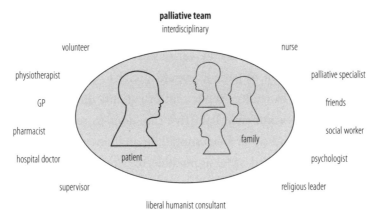

complaint the doctor's medical advice becomes urgent. All healthcare workers should have a basic knowledge of all four dimensions in order to know who to contact on a particular problem.

Although this model sounds good in theory, it doesn't always work in practice. In fact it can only work when doctors move away from the entrenched autonomous expertise or paternalistic care model. Nevertheless, it is worth pursuing as it can contribute significantly when taking major decisions. When a decision needs to be made about giving a generalised cancer patient palliative chemotherapy, or whether an advanced AIDS sufferer is benefiting from a palliative day unit, participatory decision-making is the best model. All decisions should be discussed with the patient (and possibly their family) as well as the other team members. This may seem obvious, and yet is not widely practised, leading to frustration on all sides.

Respect for the patient's beliefs

In a pluralistic society we acknowledge the co-existence of different principles and beliefs. This is equally important in the patient–healthcare professional relationship. The healthcare professional is duty bound to show respect for the patient's values and beliefs regardless of their own. If they are unable to do so, they must refer the patient to someone else. This is a fundamental human and patient right.

Horizontal cooperation at macro level

What is important for a patient at micro level is also important at macro level: the cooperation between the various care facilities. It is known that in Belgium 70 per cent of patients would prefer to be cared for at home until the very end. In reality 70 per cent of patients die in the hospital or residential care environments. Palliative care aims to respond to patients' needs and wishes, and so its focus should be on home care. It is important that the patient be allowed, as far as possible, to choose where they are cared for at each stage of their illness: at home, an alternative home environment (residential care centres), in hospital, in a palliative care unit or in a specialist palliative day unit.

Palliative care: by everyone

Palliative care is not a privilege bestowed on patients by an elite group of specialised 'dying escorts'. Dying is a normal process and almost every healthcare professional is confronted with it at some stage, and should therefore be able to offer basic palliative care. Only if confronted with a specific problem about which they lack knowledge or where the burden is too great, should the healthcare professional be able to call on 'second-line' palliative care support, also called structured or specialist palliative care (see p. 35).

Palliative care is so much more than terminal care

The current definition of palliative care rightly introduces this advice as early as possible in the illness. The expertise of palliative teams should not be restricted to the terminal phase of the disease. Moreover, during active treatment such as chemotherapy there is usually a need for additional support in the form of pain control or psychosocial care. The concept of palliative care includes both early *supportive care* in parallel with palliative medicine (see p. 15–16) for an incurable disease as well as *terminal care* for a patient in the final phase of their illness. This care in the final phase of a patient's life is referred to as 'palliative terminal care' in the Netherlands. Unfortunately, in reality the palliative teams are too often notified too late, by which stage there is little they can contribute, other than giving advice during the dying phase. Bereavement for loved ones can be difficult. Palliative care therefore includes supportive care, terminal care and bereavement care (see p. 23).

Palliative care and euthanasia

According to the international definition of palliative care, death is neither brought forward nor delayed. This means that euthanasia – the intentional ending of a life at the explicit request of the patient – is not part of palliative care.

We know from history that both palliative care and euthanasia have their fervent supporters and opponents. This does not, however, help the patient faced with a personal choice. In neighbouring countries, the debate is equally intense. But we are not looking for polarisation between palliative care and euthanasia. It also does not make sense that euthanasia should be considered as good palliative care, as some would like. This would imply that palliative care professionals who do not want to practice euthanasia – which is their absolute right – cannot provide good quality palliative care. Palliative care is about *care* for incurable patients with limited life expectancy and also for their families. Euthanasia is the patient's clear *choice* to terminate their life.

In an ideal health system many patients would choose palliative care. Some would prefer euthanasia without palliative support. Others would opt for euthanasia while receiving palliative care. The reality, however, is still far from ideal. Far too many patients experience degrading deaths. This provides a strong argument in favour of discussing palliative care and end-of-life decisions including euthanasia as early as possible in the illness. After all, it is a patient's fundamental right to be informed of all available treatments and decisions so that they can make informed choices. This is also known as advance care planning (see pp. 171 and 189).

For the reasons mentioned above, a 'Dignified Life's End' academic chair was created by deMens.nu – a liberal humanist organisation – in mid-2011 at the Vrije Universiteit Brussel (VUB, Free University of Brussels).

It is a unique post, and worldwide the first time all options relating to end of life decisions (including euthanasia) are given equal value (www. waardiglevenseinde.eu). The author of this book is the current chair.

Optimal palliative care cannot alleviate all the suffering of terminally ill patients

Even in the UK, the birthplace of palliative care, it is not possible to alleviate all suffering at the end of life. It is for this reason that Elizabeth Dare, a feisty, independent 76-year-old woman suffering from colon cancer made a reconnaissance visit to Brussels in Belgium in May 2014. She wanted to investigate the possibility of euthanasia and whether it would be available to her. She then returned to her old life in Kent, reassured in the knowledge that medically she qualified for euthanasia. The Belgian Euthanasia Law does not require Belgian nationality but it insists on a good doctor–patient relationship to prevent 'euthanasia tourism'. At the beginning of July her condition deteriorated rapidly and the local palliative care team was called in. Despite good care, her situation was no longer tenable: she couldn't swallow, was vomiting blood and in excruciating pain. She requested an ambulance to bring her to Brussels. Given that her sons could not help her – assisting a suicide is an offence in the UK, punishable by up to 14 years in prison – a friend from the South of France flew to join her and made arrangements for her to leave for Belgium. She died just before her departure on Sunday 13 July 2014 at home in Ashford in a way that she never wanted.

Ironically, just a few days later, on 18 July, Lord Falconer's Assisted Dying Bill was the subject of a marathon debate in the House of Lords. The bill passed its Second Reading uncontested, but there is still a long way to go before it can be ratified as law. But even if this law had already been in force in the UK, it would not have helped Elizabeth Dare. The Assisted Dying Bill stipulates that a doctor may make the lethal drugs available to a terminally ill patient (with life expectancy of less than 6 months; see p. 166). The patient must be able to self-administer, something which Elizabeth Dare would not have been able to do orally as she could no longer swallow, but which may well have been able to have been done in another way. Fortunately this distinction is not required in the Belgian Euthanasia Law (see p. 148).

Palliative care and bereavement

Palliative care concerns the patient and their family. It makes sense, therefore, that supporting bereaved family members is part of palliative care. Bereavement care can be given by palliative nurses trained to recognise complex grief symptoms and refer family members to specialist bereavement counsellors if necessary.

*   *   *

In conclusion, here's the abbreviated definition of palliative care from the Belgian law of 14 June 2002 on palliative care:

> Everything involved in providing care to patients with life-threatening illnesses that no longer respond to curative treatment. Multidisciplinary care is essential for patients at the end of their lives on a physical, psychological, social and moral level. The main goal of palliative care is to provide the patient and his entourage with the best possible quality of life and to offer maximum autonomy. Palliative care is aimed at optimising the patient's quality of life, and that of his family, in the time that he has left.

2 The development of palliative care in Flanders*

It is innately human to comfort and provide care to those suffering from cancer, particularly those close to death. Yet what seems self-evident at an individual, personal level has, by and large, not guided policy at the level of institutions in this country.

Kathleen Foley

Bottom up: the fledgling initiative stemming from basic need

Palliative care or hospice care didn't just happen by chance in the United Kingdom in the middle of the last century. It grew up in response to the appalling conditions at the time in English hospitals, where cancer patients sometimes died.

Healthcare in the UK has its own structure, which has resulted in two-tier medicine: the Government-funded NHS (National Health Service), with waiting lists, and more accessible but expensive private medicine. Hence the British tradition of charitable fundraising by local communities, particularly for palliative care. Welfare foundation offices or charity shops are to be found on every corner: Cancer Research, Marie Curie Foundation, British Heart Foundation, St Christopher's Hospice etc. Much of the care for incurable cancer patients is funded in this way.

---

* Flanders, the Dutch-speaking part of Belgium, contains 60 per cent of the population, around 6,600,000 of the 11,100,000 Belgians.

Dame Cicely Saunders, a nurse who later went on to study medicine, was to become the 'face' of palliative care. In 1967 she founded St Christopher's Hospice in London, one of the first hospices for terminal cancer patients. Hospices are small-scale, patient-oriented 'homes' often connected with a hospital. Terminal patients, and sometimes even their families, can stay there day and night until the very end. In addition to the professional care, the patient and their family are supported by a host of volunteers. Hospice comes from the Latin word 'hospitium' or 'residence for terminal patients'. They have also been described as 'dying houses' or 'guest houses'. In Flanders they are now commonly referred to as 'residential units', 'palliative units' or simply 'units'. The impact of these hospices on the development of palliative care in the UK was so great that, especially in the early days, the term 'palliative care' and 'hospice care' were taken to mean the same thing.

Palliative care came to the European mainland much later.

In 1980 the non-profit organisation Continuing Care was set up in Brussels by Joan Jordan. She was of British descent and married to a Belgian who had incurable cancer. She soon realised that palliative care in Belgium was not as available as in the UK. She also used Continuing Care to raise awareness and funds. Then in 1985, Chantal Couvreur joined the association and they were able to provide palliative care at home.

Subsequently there has been a fundamental difference between the evolution of palliative care in Belgium and in the UK; Belgium can be considered the leader in palliative care on mainland Europe.

In the first instance, palliative care came to Belgium later than the UK, a reaction to the explosive rise of medical technology in the 1970s. The new technology demanded such attention that it drew the focus away from the seriously ill patient.

In addition, it was then clear that the focus of palliative care should be in the home. After all, most people (70 per cent) prefer to be cared for at home until they die. In reality, more than 70 per cent die in hospitals and care homes, only a quarter at home. This gave rise to 'palliative home-care teams' in various areas. The first, Omega, was set up in 1988 by Lisette Custermans, a psychiatric nurse attached to the Faculty of Medicine at the

VUB and a former active member of Continuing Care. At the end of 2013, the team's twenty-fifth anniversary was celebrated at the Royal Flemish Theatre in Brussels. In 1990, Lisette Custermans founded the umbrella organisation the Flemish Terminal Care Federation, renamed the Flanders Palliative Care Federation (Federatie Palliatieve Zorg Vlaanderen) in 1993. At the time, the much needed financial support was sourced through fairs, barbecues, service clubs and predominantly the national Kom op tegen Kanker (United Against Cancer) initiative.

Study trips: From the UK to Auschwitz

When palliative care was first introduced in Belgium I, together with Thierry Van Calster and Tony De Bondt (see p. 2) organised various study trips to England and Scotland. The aim was to refine our knowledge of pain and symptom control and psychosocial reception, and to compare the organisational aspects of palliative care. We had the honour of meeting Dame Cicely Saunders herself. A strong social bond, which some of them have maintained, developed between the participants. Reference is still made to these trips today, and there are regular calls for the initiative to be reintroduced. Belgium today, in contrast to other countries on the European mainland, has benefited from excellent professional palliative care for twenty-five years and also has more than ten years' experience with transparent euthanasia requests and respect for patients' rights. Some aspects of palliative care, such as pain and symptom control, are now very well known in Belgium. For this reason, when choosing a new study trip we decided to focus on existential suffering. As people approach the end of their lives, they are constantly confronted with questions about the meaning of life, loss, (loss of) power, self-reflection, dependency and self-determination, finiteness and, above all, worthlessness.

My good friend Lydia Chagoll, an honorary doctor at the VUB for her commitment to human rights, suggested a study trip to Auschwitz, the Nazi extermination camp. Lydia is Jewish and is a renowned filmmaker, writer and artist. She was imprisoned in Japanese concentration camps as a child and a large part of her family was gassed in Auschwitz. For the past forty years Lydia has been an official guide at Auschwitz-Birkenau, the place that perfectly symbolises a degrading (undignified) end of life.

It seemed like a good opportunity to combine her experience with a study trip. At the beginning of October 2014, approximately eighty healthcare professionals (doctors, nurses, psychologists) travelled to Auschwitz to exchange views on the problem of existential suffering and to clarify semantic confusion. The study trip was, as expected, captivating, and highly appreciated by the participants. The attitude of the healthcare professionals present was that they would now treat vulnerable patients and their existential fear with more attention and empathy. Fundamentalist opponents of euthanasia heard about this trip and informed a number of European news editors. Several sensation-seeking journalists published articles about the trip without any respect for or understanding of its purpose.

Another Belgian pioneer worth mentioning is Sister Leontine. She is a nurse who subsequently, just like Cicely Saunders in the UK, qualified as a doctor – Dr Debuysschere. After her retirement as Director of St John's Hospital, Brussels in 1990 she founded the first palliative care unit, with 12 beds.

Top down: fledgling initiatives from the Government

In 1991, the socialist Philippe Busquin, then Minister of Social Affairs, gave a number of palliative care initiatives the opportunity to conclude financial conventions with the national social security service. This meant that some palliative care initiatives (which meet certain conditions) would be recognised by the Government, and that their services would be fully state funded, and therefore free of charge for the patients. Although it amounted to little more than a symbolic sum of just over €6 million for the whole of Belgium, it was the first step in the recognition of palliative care. It also led to the first palliative support teams being set up in a number of hospitals and some care homes. This continued until 1999, when the 'Busquin experiment' budgets were revised and increased to provide home-care teams – 15 in Flanders, 24 in Belgium – with reasonable funding. Nearly ten long years after the days of the village fairs, the press conferences, the lobbying, and most of all a lot of frustration and burnout among pioneers of palliative care, finally the initiative was properly funded. Despite the frustrations, it was a hugely rewarding period, because it was a time of intense cohesion without the restriction of different ideologies and their structures.

The 'network' period, the amending of the Government conventions and the birth of palliative day-care units

The then Flemish Minister Wivina Demeester (Christian Democrats) was intent on doing something about the precarious situation of palliative home care. In 1995 she asked the 15 home-care teams in Flanders to organise a so-called palliative care 'network' in their region, and she provided a fixed sum of money per network to appoint a regional 'coordinator'. Given that many of the networks at the time barely had the resources for patient support, this 'network' grant was frequently used for patient care.

In 1997, I opened the first day centre for palliative care support (Topaz) with support from the VUB's academic hospital – the University Hospital Brussels). Before setting it up I made several research trips to the UK for inspiration. The concept behind Topaz is ultimately based on the London Lighthouse; an inspirational palliative day-care unit for terminal AIDS patients in West London, supported by, among others, Elton John. Coda Hospice, a similar day-care centre, opened in the same year. The third day-care centre, Bethanië, was opened some time later by Sister Leontine. The University Hospital Brussels preferred to invest in this new concept rather than in a residential unit, for two main reasons: on the one hand to introduce the fourth model of palliative care in Belgium, and on the other to propose a new shelter for serious chronic illnesses. With the exponential ageing of the population, it is time to invest in patient-friendly and financially appealing alternatives. In 2002, ten palliative day-care units signed a convention with the Government.

It was also in 1997 that all residential care homes were required to be able to provide a palliative function. This is broadly defined to include all activities designed to support the treatment and care of incurably ill patients. In 1999 it became obligatory for all hospitals to set up a 'mobile support team' for the palliative function. Since 1997, there have been 360 dedicated palliative beds in Belgium, divided between the different palliative units.

The 2000–3 palliative care policy: Magda Aelvoet (Greens) and Frank Vandenbroucke (Socialists)

The formation of the purple-green (Liberals–Socialists–Greens) coalition in 1999 injected fresh energy into the healthcare sector. For the first time palliative care felt that it was being taken seriously as an equal partner. In addition, the global budget for structured palliative care doubled: an additional €37 million or so per year. New measures were introduced, such as the granting of 'palliative leave' to cater for the 'paradox of home care', that most people die in the hospital when they would rather die at home.

Moreover, a patient's home care is often more expensive than hospital care for the patient, although hospitals are generally perceived to be more expensive for society.

The Belgian law on palliative care

On 14 June 2002, just two weeks after euthanasia was legalised in Belgium on 28 May, the law on palliative care was passed. The laws provided for the formation of two evaluation bodies: the Federal Control and Evaluation Commission, created by the law on euthanasia of 28 May 2002 (Royal Decree 2 August 2002) and the Federal Assessment Unit on Palliative Care (Royal Decree 3 February 2003).

As yet, the law on palliative care has little content and remains rather vague. It is, nevertheless, very important because for the first time the right to palliative care is legally recognised.

The Federal Assessment Unit established by law is required to evaluate the needs and the quality of palliative care every two years and report its findings to the legislative chambers. Alongside the Euthanasia and Palliative Care Laws, 2002 also saw the introduction in Belgium of the very important Patients' Rights Law.

3 Countries with euthanasia legislation

A reason to live
Makes almost anything bearable

Friedrich Nietzsche

In parallel with the rise of palliative care in Belgium there was a rise in support for the right to self-determined death, or euthanasia. The Association pour le Droit de Mourir dans la Dignité (Association for the Right to Die with Dignity, ADMD) was founded in the French-speaking part of Belgium in 1982. Then in 1983 Leon Favyts founded the pluralistic association Recht op Waardig Sterven (Right to Die with Dignity, RWS) in Antwerp, Flanders. The right to self-determination was central to both organisations. In addition to fighting for euthanasia to be legalised, they also opposed any form of therapeutic persistence, insisting that the patient should be involved in every decision concerning the end of their life. Both associations agreed that palliative care was a valid alternative to futile medical treatment, but that it should never be forced on the patient. They also created a 'negative' will (formerly referred to as a 'living will') in which people specify any treatment which they choose not to receive in certain circumstances. This document was the predecessor of 'advance care planning' or ACP (see pp. 171 and 189). In fact these associations foresaw the 2002 Patients' Rights Law.

Today the document is available free from various organisations, including LEIF (see p. 171).

During this same period, the first proposals for euthanasia legislation were submitted (in 1984, 1986 and 1988). These were later followed by further proposals (in 1993, 1994, 1995 and 1996). Despite all this reflection, no action was taken since the topic had become 'unmentionable' under the dominant Christian Democrats. Regular debates were held on the subject of euthanasia. The palliative movement itself attracted little debate. They were two separate worlds. In addition, the political environment at the time was not conducive to legislative initiatives. The debates were therefore largely theoretical and dealt with questions such as whether or not there would be a demand for euthanasia, and whether it would be ethically justifiable to provide it.

The subject was even shunned in the palliative sector: 'It does not belong in the world of palliative care.' In addition, many believed that optimal administration of palliative care would result in the 'negligible number' of requests for euthanasia disappearing altogether.

The public debate was further stimulated by the incisive, autobiographical film *Minder dood dan de anderen* (*Less Dead than the Others*, 1993) by Frans Buyens, Lydia Chagoll's partner (see p. 26), in which he narrates the accidental death of his brother, his father's suffering from lung cancer and how his mother (also suffering from cancer) was euthanised.

In 1995, Prof. Hugo Van den Enden, moral philosopher at Ghent University, published his book *Ons Levenseinde Humaniseren* (*Humanising Death*) which provides a sharp and insightful look at all possible end-of-life decisions. It is without a doubt a must-read book on the subject for any Dutch speaker. A fully revised edition was published in 2004.

In 1997, at the request of the Chamber and Senate, the Belgian Advisory Committee on Bioethics formulated an initial opinion on the desirability of a legal framework to cover euthanasia. This first opinion was limited to patients in desperate situations who are capable of expressing themselves. The pluralist composition of the committee meant that a unanimous decision was unlikely, and yet the reflection process was very important. The term 'euthanasia' was finally clearly defined as 'the intentional termination of a person's life, at his request, by a third party'. In this, the definition is completely in line with the Dutch concept of 'euthanasia'. Henceforth the historical and emotionally charged use of expressions such as euthanasia at the request of family, euthanasia of newborns, euthanasia for economic reasons, and euthanasia for dementia patients could no longer be used. Anyone involved in the debate was forced to accept that euthanasia had to be specifically requested by the patient themselves. The reaction among the foreign press to Belgium's Euthanasia Law and its implications is largely based on the broader interpretation of the term. In many countries, such as the USA, euthanasia means the termination of a person's life *with or without* them having specifically requested it.

In 1999, the Advisory Committee delivered their opinion on the termination of the life of a person unable to express themselves. This proposal introduced the notion of the 'advance declaration of one's living will'. Certain members of the committee also pushed for regulation on other decisions relating to the dying process such as palliative sedation, increased pain relief for intolerable pain, life termination without consent, assisted suicide and stopping or not starting treatment.

On 2 February 1999 Socialists Fred Erdman and Roger Lallemand submitted a draft proposal for legislation. Despite the intense social debate this provoked, it did not result in legislation.

In the parliamentary elections on 13 June 1999, the Christian Democrats lost power for the first time in decades and ended up in opposition. The purple–green majority coalition of Liberals, Socialists and Greens was determined to promote 'laws and regulations on relevant issues in a modern, democratic and pluralist society', such as euthanasia. Once again proposals for a Euthanasia Bill were submitted by several politicians.

Finally on 20 December 1999 six senators of the majority parties submitted three joint legislative proposals: one on euthanasia, one on the setting up of a Federal Control and Evaluation Commission on the Application of the Euthanasia Law, and one on palliative care.

The bill proposed by the majority parties was clearly inspired by the Socialist proposal originally submitted by Erdman and Lallemand: euthanasia may only be practised on patients whose medical condition is hopeless and whose physical suffering is unbearable, but in addition it would be available for psychic suffering, for non-terminal patients and by means of a pre-established testament (advance declaration). In the hope that this bill would reach a broad social consensus, 40 witnesses were invited in the spring of 2000 to a series of public hearings organised by the United Senate Committees for Justice and Social Affairs. These public debates were very intense. Never before had there been such an extended period of collective reflection about suffering, dying and palliative care. This ended with a general consensus on the importance of good palliative support. The majority parties had hoped that these hearings would get the Christian Democrats on side, but the opposition remained faithful to its position. More than six hundred amendments were made during the discussion of the articles in the bill.

Meanwhile, outside the legislative chambers, the debates also became very heated and were closely monitored by the media. Representatives from the palliative care sector joined the public debate, not all of them completely committed to intellectual integrity. Others, myself included, were concerned that this would lead to euthanasia being applied without first considering all the possibilities offered by palliative care. Prof. Bert Broeckaert of the Catholic University of Leuven and Ethics Adviser at the Flanders Palliative Care Federation (at the time I was president of this federation) therefore introduced the concept of a palliative 'filter'. He proposed that every patient requesting euthanasia be legally required to attend a consultation with a palliative care team. Despite sharing the concerns expressed by Bert Broeckaert, I became convinced that this would only serve to weigh down the procedure. Of course a patient must be made aware of – not be subjected to – all the possibilities that palliative care can offer before opting for euthanasia. However, it is up to the attendant doctor to decide whether he or she is sufficiently competent to provide this information without recourse to a palliative consultation. Adopting the above reasoning would mean that a compulsory consultation with a psychologist, a religious leader or liberal humanist could also be required.

Some care institutions and doctors took (and continue to take) a much narrower view of the palliative 'filter': not only should the patient be aware of all possible palliative options but they should also have tried them before any request for euthanasia could be honoured.

In the period leading up to the law, many prosecutors were uneasy. There was an unprecedented amount of reporting about doctors and nurses involved in the illegal termination of life. Even pain management in the context of good palliative care was sometimes described as euthanasia, thus compromising the practice. This was undoubtedly due to the fact that a legislative initiative was now a real possibility.

On 25 October 2001 the legislative proposals of the majority parties were approved by the entire Senate. On 28 May 2002, after a vote in the plenary, Belgium, like the Netherlands, had its own Euthanasia Law. Two weeks later, the law on palliative care was passed.

The Euthanasia Law came into force on 23 September 2002, three months after publication in the Official Gazette (22 June 2002).

Both laws provided for in the creation of evaluation bodies, as already mentioned, respectively the Belgian Federal Control and Evaluation Commission (commonly known as the Federal Euthanasia Commission) and the Belgian Federal Assessment Unit on Palliative Care.

4 Structured palliative care

Every policy should have the aim of putting people first.

Bill Clinton

The palliative care sector has always campaigned for the incurably ill to be treated in the environment of their choice; most would choose their own homes. It also believes that all healthcare providers should have a basic knowledge of palliative care, particularly in the fields of pain and symptom control and psychological and spiritual guidance.

For the average healthcare provider palliative care can, at times, be either too time consuming or too complex. In certain cases they will therefore request help from the so-called structured palliative care team or even transfer the care of the patient to these teams. The structured palliative care model forms part of second-line care and as such is subsidised by the Government and intended to provide support for patients with incurable illnesses during the final weeks or possibly months of their lives. In contrast to the above, 'palliative culture' focuses on incurable life-threatening illnesses, which are not necessarily terminal (see below). Of course palliative teams play an important role in this context, primarily in an advisory role, which inevitably leads to many bottlenecks.

It is important that the palliative team should be consulted for its opinion. Unfortunately this is not as obvious as it seems. Doctors and other healthcare professionals who don't know enough about the benefits of palliative care 'don't know what they don't know', and will therefore refrain from asking for supportive advice. As a result palliative teams, in addition to providing expert advice, also have to expend a lot of energy convincing their co-workers of their value, making the threat of burnout very real. It would be naive to think that palliative care teams would become redundant if all professional care givers were competent in dealing with end-of-life care. Dr Derek Doyle, a Scottish doctor with an incredible sense of humour, and a pioneer in palliative care who founded the International Association for Hospice and Palliative Care, and received on 9 July 2014 the award of Honorary Doctor of Science from the University of Glasgow, told me in 1997 that the watchdog role of structured palliative care remains imperative. Without it, futile therapeutic persistence will not diminish as long as medical training in most medical facilities focuses exclusively on healing.

Structured palliative care models

Currently there are four palliative care models that receive support from the Government. They are based on similar models in the UK, namely palliative home-care teams, mobile support teams in hospitals and their equivalent in residential care homes, hospices and day-care units.

In addition, Flanders has been divided in 15 regions (so-called networks) since 1995. The aim is that in each region the palliative care models, traditional healthcare providers, and care facilities – home care, residential care homes, hospitals, voluntary bodies and so on – all work together to provide optimal care for palliative patients in the environment of their choice.

1. Palliative home-care teams

A home-care team consists mostly of experienced nurses who attend exclusively to terminal patients, for which they receive special training. They do not replace classic traditional home care – GP, district nurse, physiotherapist etc. – but complete it. It is not an easy task, as they often have to convince the traditional team of the added value of palliative care as well as take over certain aspects of treatment in which the non-specialist carer is less adept. This requires sensitivity. The average GP probably treats five terminal patients per year. This does not provide them with extensive experience in palliative care. On the other hand, they have broad medical knowledge and are well acquainted with the patient and their family. Palliative teams need to strike a balance between giving advice and acknowledging the doctor as having the final medical responsibility. Relations with the hardworking nurses are also not always easy. They often think that the palliative teams have a cushy job because they can 'spend lots of time with the patient' while they are being run off their feet. The emotional drain of always dealing with terminal patients and their families is often forgotten.

The above illustrates the importance of interdisciplinary work. Optimal care can only be achieved with mutual respect between the different disciplines. In this way, the GP and district nurse will be convinced that with the help of palliative care a patient can be treated at home longer, even until the end.

There are 15 home-care teams in Flanders, one per palliative network. The teams consist of between two and eight specialist nurses, depending on the size of the region, administrative help and at least one part-time GP with palliative experience. Some teams also receive support from a psychologist.

After approval from the attendant physician, the team may be called upon, for which they will be paid a flat rate. Home-care teams are available day and night and their services are completely free for the patient.

2a. Palliative support teams in hospitals

Palliative support teams in hospitals – also referred to as mobile support teams or simply support teams – must consist of at least a part-time physician with palliative experience, a part-time qualified nurse and a part-time clinical psychologist. Each hospital receives a subsidy for this purpose, and is required to establish a team. Hospitals also explicitly opted to include a medical specialist in the team to be able to negotiate on the same level as other specialists on the pros and cons of different treatments and examinations.

The primary role of the hospital support teams, as with the home-care teams, is advisory. They provide bedside training for fellow healthcare colleagues and only take over the care responsibility if specifically asked.

These teams can also be involved in discharging patients so that they can return home. In doing so they will have to contend with the hospital's 'pseudo-security' – 'a patient cannot go home with a drip' (why not?) and 'the patient is in danger of dying en route' (surely the same threat is present in the hospital?). In addition to their role of ombudsman, these teams also provide a point of contact for extra-mural staff. They can be notified if a palliative patient has been hospitalised for a specific problem, and thus save the patient from again being subjected to the diagnosis and treatment mill.

Any move to reduce futile therapeutic persistence should start in hospitals. Hospital teams are well placed to open negotiations on incurability, suffering and dying in hospitals; the isolated nature of palliative care units makes them less so.

These palliative teams must be given the opportunity to prove their worth. This requires that hospital management not only allows but also actively supports palliative care. The role of these teams is only advisory, and given the energy with which illnesses are diagnosed and treated in general hospitals, their impact is not immediately obvious. Many specialists hide behind diagnosis and treatment as the primary mission of a hospital. This type of environment is not conducive to spontaneous examinations and interventions, and as a result the palliative team is often called in too late when there is time only to organise a quick return home or to help extreme terminal patients die an 'elegant' death.

In addition, palliative care in university or larger hospitals is often considered to be in direct 'competition' with clinical trials (as if they were mutually exclusive). And yet, a patient who wants to test an experimental drug also has the right to good physical and psychosocial support. In private hospitals the problem of doctors' funding arises. They are only paid for what they themselves do.

Patients and their families should all be aware that they can always ask for advice from the hospital's mobile support teams.

2b. Palliative care in residential care homes

Residential care homes need to be able to offer palliative care. Quite how this is to be achieved is less obvious. With limited subsidies it may be possible to employ a palliative expert or to offer training to staff members. The aim of the palliative role is to prevent a resident from being taken to hospital in an ambulance with sirens blaring for pointless treatment, only to die a lonely death.

3. Hospices

A hospice is a replacement home for patients with limited family care or for whom the burden of home care is too great. In Belgium there are 360 palliative beds that are divided between palliative units. One unit has between six and twelve beds. They can be incorporated into the hospital architecture, for example the Sister Leontine palliative unit in St John's Hospital in Brussels, or be separate, like the Coda Hospice in Wuustwezel. The medical responsibility lies with a specialist, although there are a few exceptions. General practitioners are encouraged to follow up on their patients at the hospice. The patient is surrounded by healthcare providers such as nurses, a psychologist, a religious leader, a lay counsellor, a physiotherapist and volunteers. Families are also welcome.

In the past, hospices were considered places where terminally ill patients were sent to die. Today, however, just as in the UK, they are perceived more and more as temporary care places to resolve difficult problems or as respite for the family and other carers, giving them some breathing space.

Palliative units are sometimes described as 'sheltered employment' since neither patients nor healthcare providers are forced to compete with futile therapeutic persistence – palliative care is the sole focus. Nevertheless, the impact of being permanently confronted with death should not be underestimated. There is definite solidarity within the unit but the process is 'socially isolated'. The environment is different from a hospital; here palliative patients are interspersed with recovering patients. They help to dispel the taboo around death and dying.

Due to the very specific nature of these units, patients are more or less forced to come to terms with their own death. Patients who are in denial will be difficult to treat unless they have been (forcibly) informed of their prognosis. Sister Leontine once described her unit as an 'experimental lab' set up to provide healthcare workers with quick, sound training in terminal care, and it remains a valuable alternative for patients without family or other forms of care. Nevertheless there is not the same 'density' of palliative beds in Belgium as there is in the UK. Priority has been given to palliative home care, particularly in Flanders.

4. Day-care units

Day-care units are the most recent and least known model in Belgium. For this reason they will be discussed in greater depth.

The first day-care units for palliative patients were established in the UK. There are currently approximately two hundred and fifty operational day centres with waiting lists. In Belgium this would translate to the equivalent of between forty and forty-five day-care units. The first day-care units in Belgium were set up towards the end of the nineties. The first, Topaz, was, founded by the University Hospital Brussels in Wemmel, closely followed by Coda in Wuustwezel as a private initiative, and Bethanië in Brussels attached to St John's Hospital. An experimental government subsidy for day-care units was included in the 2000–3 Palliative Care Policy introduced by ministers Aelvoet and Vandenbroucke. In 2002, 10 day-care units signed a convention.

As already mentioned, in contrast to the UK, Flanders gave precedence to palliative home care. Day-care units fit this model perfectly. Proportion-ally, more day-care units than there are in the UK would have to be set up in the long term.

Day-care units are the perfect bridge between hospitals and home care. On the one hand they accelerate the return home from hospital, and on the other they mean that patients can also stay at home longer.

Day-care units can provide the perfect solution for long-term patients torn between the safety of the hospital and the desire to return home. Patients can even visit day-care units sporadically during their hospitalisation, thus rendering their discharge from the hospital almost seamless, with the reassurance that they are supported even at home. Once home, the patients can continue to visit the day-care units. The burden for the family and other carers is lessened and there is no need for the seriously ill to be continually hospitalised. Day-care units give the patient 'a day out' and the carer 'a day off'.

The advantage of day-care units is that the patient has social contact as well as being able to receive treatment for which they would otherwise have to go to a hospital: blood transfusions, bathing using a hoist, psychological support. Everything is possible and nothing is obligatory. There is a light, relaxed atmosphere while the professionals remain attentive to any physical and psychological needs. Day-care units are complementary to home care with a focus on 'living'. Traditional home carers are also welcome: the physiotherapist for revalidation exercises, the district nurse to treat wounds, the family doctor for an incision and drainage, for example.

Treatment by palliative home-care teams or in palliative units usually lasts weeks, sometimes months, whereas patients in day-care units usually have longer life expectancy: a further indication that palliative does not necessarily mean terminal.

The distinction seems artificial and in practice the transition between curative, palliative and terminal is often unclear. Cancer patients with recurrent and uncertain prognoses can enjoy a temporary break in a day-care unit. AIDS patients who are struggling to comply with their therapy may be given a new lease of life following a visit to a day-care unit and be re-motivated to continue their antiviral treatment and reintegrate into society.

Due to the presence of qualified healthcare professionals, day-care units may also contribute to a reduction in futile therapeutic persistence (see Chapter 15). They allow for informal discussions on the usefulness of active treatment. The net result is that patients feel supported and healthcare providers are given additional support. Hence it might be better to call them 'supportive day-care units'.

Traditional healthcare professionals need time to adjust to the concept of a 'day-care unit patient'. The traditional expectations of medicine still predominate: curative treatment, and only when this is no longer possible the patient is 'left' to the palliative care teams. Between the two extremes of cure/healing and terminal care is the (huge) grey area of palliation, namely the area of 'trial and error', of relapse, of emotional turmoil, of hope and despair, of research into and trying out of different treatments, of adapting to new living conditions. Day-care units, in addition to receiving already advanced patients, are perfectly suited to welcome patients from this grey area of palliation.

In addition, patients at day-care units tend to be younger – often with working partners – than those cared for by other palliative teams.

The recommendations of the Council of Europe (Rec. (2003) 24 of the Committee of Ministers to member states on the organisation of palliative care) are very clear: day care must be part of the healthcare package available to patients. The following quote is taken from these recommendations:

> patients may attend one or more days a week. The facilities on offer may be of a medical nature (blood transfusions, pain and symptom control, etc.), of a social nature (shower/bath), related to revalidation (physiotherapy, activity therapy), of a relaxing nature (massage) or of a non-cerebral nature (arts and crafts). They also allow the primary healthcare provider some free time.

The importance of day-care units is not to be underestimated in a changing society with less and less informal care.

The nuclear family keeps getting smaller, and often consists of two working partners. If one partner should fall seriously ill, there will be no-one to look after them during the day. In such instances, 'forced' hospitalisation could be avoided by day care.

The ageing population means that more and more people are living with chronic and often life-threatening conditions. There is therefore a need to find alternative residential care facilities; the existing care homes cannot be expanded ad infinitum.

Supportive day-care units offer the perfect alternative to counter all these obstacles.

The role of volunteers in the different palliative care models

It is not always easy for healthcare providers treating patients with life-threatening diseases, but their task would be impossible without the support and commitment of countless volunteers. Volunteers play a vital role in palliative care (even with sufficient financial resources). They do not replace, but rather complement, the work of the healthcare professional. In addition to helping the patients with innumerable activities, such as transport, preparing meals, preparing creative leisure activities, listening, 'being there', they also act as an early warning system for the healthcare professionals. And last but not least they form part of an invaluable movement in society that should accept and relate to seriously ill patients' declining health, suffering and dying.

Palliative care networks

Flanders is divided into 15 network regions corresponding to the areas covered by the 15 palliative home-care teams, with populations varying from two hundred thousand to in excess of nine hundred thousand. Each region receives subsidies from both the Federal Government and the Flemish Community. Each network has at least a coordinator and a part-time clinical psychologist. Other larger networks also have people in charge of training, bereavement care, volunteers, administration etc.

Anyone can consult the networks for practical information about palliative care. They form the 'cement' between the palliative care facilities in the region and hospitals, residential care centres, doctors (GPs), nurses, family assistance etc. They can act as a mediator for the palliative patient whenever they have a problem of any kind. The networks are also responsible for providing training to both professionals and volunteers, and to raise awareness about dying and death.

Other palliative facilities

The idea behind these provisions is to facilitate palliative home care and to cater for the 'paradox of home care'. Patients wishing to apply for funding must acquire a 'palliative' status.

1. Fixed allowance for palliative patients

A 'palliative patient' who wishes to stay at home is entitled to an allowance of approximately €600 per month (maximum two months). All that is required is that their GP complete the relevant form.

2. Palliative leave

Any person wishing to stay at home to care for a terminal patient (it does not have to be a family member) is entitled to palliative leave (one month, twice).

3. Home nursing allowance and refund of the patient's contribution to doctors' and physiotherapists' fees.

Palliative patients are entitled to home nursing that would normally be reserved for care dependant patients, using the home nursing allowance. In practice this means that the patient does not have to pay the doctor for a home visit, it is free for the patient. The same applies to physiotherapists.

Non-governmental support for palliative care

In addition to regular funding from the Government, some institutions make annual appeals for renewable funding or via projects. These private and local initiatives – such as service clubs, organising benefit concerts, barbecues etc. – are desperately needed, just as they are in the UK.

It would be fair to ask why it is that end-of-life care in a modern society should have to be funded with the proceeds from charitable initiatives. In this respect Belgium is relatively lucky compared to other countries.

Flanders Palliative Care Federation

The Federatie Palliatieve Zorg Vlaanderen (Flanders Palliative Care Federation) is a union for palliative care initiatives. Certain initiatives have left the union as a result of a difference in vision and ethics.

The Belgian Federal Palliative Care Assessment Unit

This committee is the counterpart of the Federal Euthanasia Commission. It is composed of representatives working in the sector. Their task is to produce a bi-annual report on the evolution and obstacles of palliative care in Belgium which is submitted to the legislative chambers. The first report was delivered in 2005.

5 Delivering bad news*

A sharp mind is necessary to speak well, a good listener requires only intelligence.

André Gide

The patient and their family are the central focus of healthcare. The patient must therefore be involved in all decisions regarding their health from the beginning of treatment, in order that the patients' autonomy and identity is respected.

Once the diagnosis has been established, an experienced doctor will very quickly be able to determine whether the condition is curable (curative medicine), is no longer curable but can be kept under control (palliative medicine), or whether the disease has entered the final phase and palliative terminal care is necessary. The distinction is not clear to the uninformed patient because the same tests and treatments may be used in both the curative and palliative phases. Failure on the part of the healthcare professional to inform the patient adequately can lead to frustration for the patient and their family because of different expectations. The worst example would be a doctor wanting to test only the potential side-effects of a new drug on an incurable cancer patient who mistakenly believes that there is a chance they might be cured.

---

* With thanks to Manu Keirse.

Knowledge is power. (Francis Bacon)

For no other reason than respect for their autonomy, the patient has the right to be involved in decisions concerning their own health. The recent Belgian Patients' Rights Law sends an important message to healthcare providers about their attitudes towards their patients.

Informed choices are based on comprehensive, reliable information. The doctor should therefore inform the patient, in a language that they understand, of all the choices available to them. Doctors often subtly promote their own personal preference and pay little or no attention to other alternatives, in order to influence the patient. This is wrong. The information should be objective and complete and in no way influenced by personal preference, ignorance of alternatives, economic motives or scientific studies. It is known but also understandable that medical specialists recommend a treatment with which they are familiar and trust: a surgeon will look at a surgical solution, a radiation oncologist will be inclined to opt for radiation; a palliative doctor will prefer palliative sedation to euthanasia. But this does not mean that it is the best solution for the patient. There is an urgent need for interdisciplinary dialogue in which palliative care is rightfully considered as a viable alternative in itself rather than an appendage to so-called curative treatment.

Not everyone shares the same idea of what constitutes 'quality of life'. People often make the mistake of saying 'if I were in his shoes, I wouldn't want to live'. The concept of quality of life is very personal and can only be determined through consultation with the patient.

It is important that this consultation and the provision of the right information takes place as soon as possible after the first contact in order to avoid complications later.

The whole truth and nothing but the truth?

Blurting out the truth and leaving the patient to deal with it is as traumatic as not saying anything or even lying. But between these two extremes there are a multitude of possibilities. Respect for the patient's autonomy has to be weighed up against respect for the patient as a human being.

In principle, one should never lie. A doctor who lies can then not backtrack without losing the confidence of the patient and their family. It also hinders communication with other healthcare professionals. Nevertheless, there are times when a half truth is the best option. Someone with localised breast cancer does not need to know about all possible metastases and their treatment options. In a similar way, certain information can be withheld from an incurable patient – without actively lying – depending on the patient's ability to deal with the news. This can be measured by monitoring non-verbal signs of intense anxiety such as trembling hands and by listening attentively. Information may also be gleaned by talking to bystanders such as family, friends or acquaintances: 'How have they coped with previous losses and goodbyes, such as being forced to leave a job or the death of a dear family member?'

The diagnosis and the expectations

When delivering the diagnosis, the doctor must strike a compromise between the patient's right to be informed and unnecessary disruption to a person's life. A medical practitioner has an ethical duty not to inflict psychological or physical damage (see p. 184 on medical ethics).

It is important that the doctor creates a friendly impression – a handshake, a smile, seated at eye level – and a willingness to listen. It is also a good idea to involve trusted family members or friends when communicating important information, thereby limiting the number of misunderstandings and giving the patient a sounding board with whom to discuss the information.

The initial contact with the patient should be conducted with discretion in determining how much the patient already knows or suspects, and whether they have been spoken to by a specialist or GP. It is important to respond to all of their questions in language that they understand. This requires experience. Attention seeking should not be confused with wanting to know the truth. An extremely anxious patient is liable to ask questions without actually wanting to know the answer, just to reassure themselves that the healthcare professional is committed.

There are also times when patients are unable to cope with the truth. This should be respected, and information initially withheld, but it should not be used as an excuse for failing to communicate anything. Doctors and other healthcare professionals have to be attentive at all times to verbal and non-verbal signs that the patient needs more information. Listening and observing the patient means that the information can be passed on as and when the patient is ready for it. Listening is 'actively being silent' and requires patience, concentration, discipline and analytical thinking in order – together with the non-verbal observation – to extract the implicit message that is being communicated.

When the diagnosis is life-changing, the patient needs to be given time to absorb it. It is important also to ensure that the information has been correctly understood: 'Am I making myself clear?', 'Are we on the same wavelength?' Doctors have a tendency to use too much technical jargon: 'the result of the scan is negative', 'metastasis', 'cerebral oedema'. It is well known that about half of the information is being lost on the patient. It is also important that the healthcare professional indicates that they are available to answer any questions. Doctors are concerned mainly with clinical history, whereas for the patient this is inextricably intertwined with their life story, the impact on their friends and family, on hobbies and professional activities.

If complications are expected, giving the patient a contact number can often put their mind at rest. It helps to reassure them that they are cared for and makes them feel less alone. Experience shows that patients do not abuse these gestures.

The contents of each consultation with the patient and their family should be shared with all other team members. Failure to do so can lead to irrevocable errors and cause the patient to lose confidence in their care team, with serious consequences: medical shopping, resorting to questionable alternative medicine, even deep sadness or depression.

Non-verbal communication must always echo the verbal. Patients are extremely sensitive to the body language of the healthcare professional: if they appear hesitant or evasive, this is indicative of a gloomy outlook.

Doctors are not well trained to offer help to patients who will die in the foreseeable future. When the fight to extend a person's life is lost in good circumstances, the doctor has to overcome any sense of failure and put an end to active treatment without damaging their relationship with the patient.

It is fundamentally important that this possibility be anticipated from the beginning. Once it has been established that the patient may not be cured, the doctor must be prepared to communicate this information tactfully. They will then be able to stop active treatment at any time without losing the patient's trust. The subject can be broached with comments such as 'I notice you are very weak' or 'Shall we delay the chemotherapy for the time being,' thus leaving the door open for continued treatment but with a focus on comfort therapy. Patients prefer this approach to futile unilateral treatment which ultimately leads to an inevitable breach of trust.

And yet there are still many – mostly elderly – patients for whom, despite all efforts at communication, it is all 'too much' or who would rather leave all decisions to the professionals: 'Do what you think is best for me.' This is not a reason to stop trying to paint a complete picture of the situation. It may be possible to involve the patient in the decision-making process again at a later stage.

Being placed in a situation where you are forced to make unilateral decisions brings with it the additional responsibility of respecting the patient and striving to avoid any psychological or physical damage: what would you think of an oncologist who systematically administers a toxic treatment to cancer patients, except when the patient is their own mother, in which case they halve the dose to reduce the side-effects?

Reactions to the information

Bad news often leads to frustration and anger. Healthcare professionals need to avoid the classic pitfall of taking this anger personally: the 'difficult' patient who continually makes life difficult for everyone despite receiving good physical care. It is important, at all costs, to avoid becoming aggressive in return, but to allow the patient the chance to express their helplessness and to understand.

A second reaction to bad news is an immature, infantile one, so-called regressive behaviour. Regression can be expressed through over-dependence, fastidiousness and an irrational reaction to the environment.

Another frequent response is denial. Negation is a normal defence mechanism (coping strategy) in dealing with unbearable news. Most patients are unable to face their approaching end of life consciously 24 hours a day. This reaction is no different to healthy people, who tend to live as if they are immortal. 'We can no more look directly at the sun than face our own death.'

Typically, incurable patients frequently fluctuate between periods of negation with moments of sober clarity: a patient may tell you one morning that they are looking forward to visiting Tenerife next winter, and in the afternoon that they have contacted the funeral parlour. This can be very confusing for inexperienced healthcare professionals, particularly if the patient has requested euthanasia.

Denial creates hope which is a very good antidote for anxiety. This hope can be rooted in reality, for example in the prospect of the birth of a new grandchild.

Insofar as denial is a form of self-protection in dealing with a serious illness it should be respected; there is no need to remind the patient continually of the reality of their situation. If the denial is omnipresent and proving to be harmful to the patient, there is usually an underlying reason which needs to be investigated, and corrected where possible. An example would be a terminal cancer patient who is in permanent denial because they are hoping for thirty years of life in order to re-establish contact with an estranged child.

In 1969, the American psychiatrist Elisabeth Kübler-Ross described five known emotional responses to bad news. In addition to the already mentioned aggression or anger and denial, she speaks of negotiation (haggling: 'What if the analysis of the scan is wrong?'), depression and acceptance. Not all patients pass through all stages, and not always in the same order. The above example illustrates that a patient in denial can go through different stages on the same day, switching from one emotion to the next. Few patients arrive at acceptance.

D.J. Theo Wagener, professor emeritus and oncologist at the St Radboud Hospital in Nijmegen, correctly maintains that Kübler-Ross did not list fear as an important emotional response.

Some patients also use humour as a tool for venting their emotions: 'I hope I meet a nice boy up there.' Healthcare professionals may not know how to deal with this. Caregivers who have a good sense of humour themselves can go along with it gently; otherwise it is better to remain neutral. As Sacha Guitry once said: 'You can pretend to be serious, but you can't pretend to be funny.'

What about the informed patient?

Out of respect for the individuality of the patient, all possible solutions should be explored together. This applies both to treatment and to how to respond to changes in their way of life such as losing a job or registering for a care home. Possible options should be proposed in moderation and not imposed. Frightening announcements such as 'We're going to place you in a care home' should be avoided. Again, if the patient rejects a given suggestion, it should not be taken personally but accepted with understanding, and the optimal solution researched in conjunction with the patient.

Dr Walter Baile and Dr Robert Buckman summarised the above into six steps known as the SPIKES model for delivering bad news:

S   (setting): create the right environment;
P   (perception): assess what the patient already knows;
I   (invitation): ask what the patient wants to know;
K   (knowledge): tell the patient and their close circle what they want to know;
E   (empathy): show empathy for the patient's emotional reaction;
S   (strategy): plan the next steps and the consequences.

6   Active treatment of incurable patients

A diligent doctor, too often, sees palliative patients through curative eyes

As life expectancy increases, more and more people are living with chronic health problems. Healthcare professionals need to adapt and change their focus from 'curing' to 'treating'. They also need to be discerning in their treatment; don't treat for the sake of treating, not too much and not too little, not too early and not too late. All treatment should be adapted to the patient and the new focus; prolonging the patient's life while at the same time optimising the quality of life of patients with incurable diseases (see below).

Incurable cancer patients

At least 80 per cent of patients who call on palliative care teams are cancer patients, both in Belgium and in the UK. This is probably due to the rapid decline in health of incurable cancer patients. I will therefore use the active treatment of these patients as a concrete example. The same principles also apply to other conditions, however.

What is active treatment?

The active treatment of cancer is based on curing or fighting the disease for as long as possible (palliation). In both cases, the latest medical technology is used: surgery, radiotherapy and chemotherapy. When active treatment is intended to cure the patient, it is referred to as curative medicine. Once it is no longer viable to try to cure the patient, as long as it is possible to contain the tumour, and hopefully thereby prolong the patient's life, it is known as palliative medicine or palliative therapy (see p. 15).

Despite all medical advances, most cancer patients still cannot be cured. Nevertheless, with use of the three treatment methods mentioned above, patients' lives with the disease are often extended. In many cases cancer can even be considered a chronic condition such as arthritis or heart disease.

Living with cancer, however, not only requires medical attention but can also create psychological problems; consider the burden of repeated harsh treatment and the fear of a relapse. For this reason, a new discipline known as 'psycho-oncology' has been developed. Clinical psychologist, Sabien Bauwens, from University Hospital Brussels, and Catherine Baillon, with support from the Flemish League Against Cancer (Vlaamse Liga tegen kanker), developed a very useful screening instrument known as the distress barometer to help the cancer patient communicate with the oncologist. It allows the patient in the waiting room to communicate the seriousness of their 'distress' (fear, pain, need for reassurance etc.) in just a few minutes. During the consultation, the results of the distress barometer are discussed with the patient, thus reassuring them that their problems are being listened to. It is also useful for the oncologist to obtain some insight into the degree of desperation of the patient. This helps to provide more comprehensive support for the patient. For example, the doctor looks at the scan of an incurable tumour, and is pleasantly surprised to see that it has reduced by a few millimetres in diameter thanks to active treatment. What the doctor hasn't noticed is that the patient has lost 20 kg as a result of the side-effects, which cause them to vomit continually and make them miserable.

The best way to actively beat cancer is a combination of several treatments. Surgery, radiotherapy and chemotherapy are often used in conjunction in treating malignant neoplasms.

This clearly illustrates the importance of remaining alert to the patient's physical and psychological problems during active treatment – even when there is a possibility that they will be cured – and reinforces the argument that experienced support teams should be involved as early as possible.

As a rule of thumb: 60 per cent of cured cancer patients are cured by surgical removal, 30 per cent by radiation and fewer than 10 per cent by chemotherapy.

The following is a description of the main principles and possibilities of palliative medicine used against cancer.

Given that chemotherapy, and especially its side-effects, are the most well-known, we'll begin with it.

Palliative chemotherapy

Fighting cancer with drugs, or chemotherapy

The term 'chemotherapy' was used for the first time at the beginning of last century by Paul Ehrlich to describe the treatment of infectious diseases with synthetically manufactured chemicals.

It was hoped that the immense success of antibiotics would be duplicated in fighting cancer cells. The term chemotherapy is now predominantly used to describe the treatment of cancer with chemicals (drugs).

Chemotherapy refers to drugs – cytostatics – that are harmful to rapidly dividing cells and hormones. In recent years products have been developed that target very specific biological pathways in the cancer cells and their immediate vicinity.

A very important area of research is attempting to identify substances that activate the immune system. The immune system is able to destroy cancer cells. Unfortunately, there is currently still a shortage of powerful, usable drugs.

Cytostatics

It is not difficult to find products that eradicate cancer tissue. Even distilled water is very effective in killing malignant cells grown in a research laboratory. Unfortunately, it is equally effective in eliminating normal cells. It is therefore necessary to find substances that *effectively* and *selectively* kill cancer cells without causing serious harm to normal tissue.

Antibiotics destroy bacteria but are harmless to humans. Research is being conducted to find an 'anti-cancer drug' which will act on malignant tumour cells without harming the human body.

Most anti-cancer or chemotherapeutic drugs inhibit the uncontrolled rapid division of cancer tissue preventing, or at least reducing, the growth of the tumour. Chemotherapy affects the whole body, thus reducing the spread of cancer cells. It is also referred to as 'systemic treatment'. It is therefore the most commonly used cancer treatment. On the down side, it also exposes healthy body tissue to the effects of the drug and therefore has more side-effects than surgery or radiation.

Anti-cancer drugs affect non-cancerous rapidly dividing tissue such as the cells in the oral mucosa, the oesophagus, the digestive tract, the blood-forming tissue in bone marrow, hair cells and skin cells. This explains the known side-effects such as mouth irritation, nausea, vomiting, diarrhoea or constipation, anaemia, susceptibility to infections, fatigue, baldness and skin irritation. The side-effects are the reason that chemotherapy is administered in limited doses. Higher doses would eliminate the cancer but the patient would either die or be seriously disabled due to damage to their vital organs.

Similarly to bacteria, cancer cells develop a resistance to these drugs. When a bacterial infection develops a resistant 'clone', the antibiotic needs to be changed. In the same way, a different chemotherapeutic agent needs to be used for mutated cancer cells. Doctors strive to avoid building up resistance to chemotherapy where possible by using different products simultaneously from the beginning.

Traditional anti-cancer products are referred to as cytotoxic (cell damaging) or cytostatic (cell-division blockers).

Hormonal cancer treatment

In addition to cytostatics, some malignant tumours can also be treated with hormones (see box below). Certain cancers stem from glandular tissue and often still have hormonal receptors. When these are stimulated by hormones their cell division capacity increases and therefore the growth of cancer cells also increases. Anti-hormones desensitise the hormone receptors and thus slow down cell division. Known examples are tamoxifen (Novaldex®) used in treating breast cancer, and gosereline (Zoladex®) used among others to treat advanced prostate cancer.

Hormones

Hormones are organic compounds formed and secreted by glandular cells with a regulating action. Hormones, together with the nervous system, are important for coordinating the functions of the different parts of higher living organisms. They are secreted directly into the bloodstream, from which they exert an influence on other tissues. Some work directly on the area where they are produced. Thanks to their binding and influence on specific receptors present on certain cells, they will only recognise and act upon certain 'target' tissue: the cells of the mammary gland are stimulated by oestrogen (female hormone), whereas the prostate is affected by the male hormone, testosterone. These hormones are produced respectively in the ovaries and testicles and in both sexes in the adrenal cortex, which also produces corticosteroids (such as cortisone), essential for balancing the body's water and salt levels.

Pending new treatments

In recent years, several other leads to develop anti-cancer drugs that act selectively on malignant tumours (in a similar way to the specific influence of [anti]-hormones) have been pursued. Methods are also being developed to strengthen the patient's immune system to offer more resistance to cancer cells. It is hoped that normal tissues would then remain unaffected, thereby reducing the side-effects. These drugs are not true cytotoxics but act by inhibiting a particular biological pathway in the tumour cell or its surroundings. They normally have to be taken for life, and the patient can also develop resistance to them. An example of one of these new drugs is trastuzumab (Herceptin®), a monoclonal antibody that targets the HER-

2/C-ERBB2 gene, which causes the overexpression of the tyrosine kinase growth-factor receptor, which then blocks the 'division' signal in breast cancer. Other examples are the angiogenesis inhibitors which block the renewal of blood vessels around the growing tumour, thereby reducing the number of tumour cells by depriving them of oxygen and nutrients. Other substances prevent tumours invading the surrounding tissue by hindering the degradation enzymes – the so-called proteinase inhibitors. Cancer cells not only penetrate their environment but also destroy it. Tumour cells are released into the whole body and form new cores, also called metastases. Groundbreaking results have recently been achieved by Bart Neyns and Kris Thielemans of the VUB using vemurafenib and dendritic cell therapy in the fight against skin cancer (melanoma).

These are all very promising treatments which may, in future, prove to be life-saving with minimum side-effects.

Palliative chemotherapy in incurable cancer patients

For the above-mentioned reasons, the extent of chemotherapy in the global healing of cancer is unfortunately limited. Only a maximum of 10 per cent of cured cancer sufferers owe this exclusively to chemotherapy. Fortunately cancer in children is an exception, and is frequently cured this way.

However, the frequency of incurable tumours in adults that respond to chemotherapy is on the increase, and many lives are being prolonged as a result.

Reducing the volume of the tumour also brings other irritating symptoms into check. Fixed tumours are often surrounded by inflammatory tissue and an accumulation of fluid. Chemotherapeutic agents act on the inflammatory cells (white blood cells) or disrupt the release of cytokines, thereby reducing the inflammation (see box below).

All these factors can therefore contribute to improving quality of life without necessarily prolonging it. This is done by reducing pain (relieving pressure on the organs), shortness of breath (decompression of the trachea), bowel obstruction (decompression of the intestinal cavity), and also by stabilising hypercalcaemia or other metabolic abnormalities.

It is important, in incurable patients, to ensure that the side-effects of (chemo)therapy are not worse than the discomforts and symptoms caused by the disease itself. The remedy should not be more harmful than the condition.

In some cases the side-effects are short-term, such as nausea and vomiting, bone marrow depression with anaemia and bleeding. Sometimes they are long-lasting and permanent, such as damage to the heart, hair loss, peripheral nerve degradation and hepatitis.

Deciding to use chemotherapy is not a simple exercise. In addition, the decisions are often taken in fairly emotionally charged circumstances: the patient has just learnt of their cancer diagnosis or that their tumour has again started to proliferate.

Cancer specialists or oncologists soon know whether a cancer patient can be cured using chemotherapy. In these cases the choice of action is obvious. If no cure is possible the advantages must be weighed against the disadvantages.

Doctors rely on a number of important parameters, listed in the following sections.

Side-effects: acceptable or not?

The side-effects of traditional chemotherapy drugs are well documented to help patients make informed decisions.

Short-term side-effects that are generally treatable, such as vomiting, would appear to be more acceptable than permanent damage, for example to the heart. It goes without saying that the patient must be involved in the decision-making process. A doctor cannot unilaterally decide on chemotherapy on the assumption that the patient would choose the possibility of living longer over quality of life, or vice versa.

Not all cancers are alike

Susceptibility to chemotherapy varies greatly from one cancer to another (see Table 1 below). It is important to consider this even in the palliative phase of the disease. The symptoms and manifestation of Hodgkin's Lymphoma in

---

The immune system and cytokines

The immune system in the human body attacks foreign molecules and germs and eliminates them without causing harm to the body. It consists of different cells that circulate freely through the human organism independently of each other. The immune systems responds to foreign tissue – bacteria, viruses and tumour cells – with a coordinated activation of various white blood cells such as lymphocytes, monocytes, basophils, eosinophils, but also of dendritic cells, endothelial cells, etc. It is becoming increasingly clear that these cells interact in different ways and thus regulate each other's activities.

Immune cells secrete two important proteins. The first, produced by specialised lymphocytes, acts as an antibody. Circulating antibodies were initially demonstrated in 1890.

In the seventies a second class of proteins was discovered, known as cytokines. They are secreted by certain lymphocytes (lymphokines) and monocytes (monokines). Cytokines are produced in limited quantities and cannot normally be detected in the blood. They are in fact hormones that interact with various target cells in the immune system and elsewhere. Known cytokines include *interleukin-1* (*IL-1*) which plays an important role in reacting to inflammation, *IL-2*, currently being studied in relation to AIDS and cancer, *IL-3* that stimulates blood creation, *interferon* α that slows the growth of certain tumours, *interferon* γ with antiviral properties and (cell) colony stimulating factors such as *g-csf* (G-colony stimulating factor) better known under the name Neupogen® (filgrastim), Neulasta® (pegfilgrastim) or Granocyte® (lenograstim) used to combat the reduction of certain white blood cells after chemotherapy to avoid the risk of infection. Some cytokines such as tumour necrosis factor (TNF) are assigned a role in anorexia-cachexia syndrome (see p. 98).

Further study of the immune system and its components will undoubtedly reveal new possibilities in the fight against cancer cells.

---

an incurable stage will still respond well to chemotherapy, in contrast to the symptoms caused by a mesothelioma (pleural cancer).

In addition, we know from scientific studies the probability of a given chemotherapy having an impact. This information is obtained by administering anti-cancer drugs to a series of selected patients. These patients must be fully informed about the possible consequences and risks of the experiment and give their full written consent. This is known as informed consent. It goes without saying that clinical studies are only conducted under the supervision of experienced physicians in oncological centres. The patient therefore has a better guarantee that their complaints and quality of life will be taken seriously during the study.

TABLE 1   CANCER RESPONSES TO CHEMOTHERAPY AND
            HORMONAL TREATMENT

I.   **Cancer curable by chemotherapy (even if advanced)**
     Germ cell tumours such as testicular cancers, seminomas and choriocarcinoma
     Non-Hodgkin's lymphoma (high grade)
     Hodgkin's lymphoma
     Acute lymphoblastic and myeloblastic leukemia
     Paediatric tumours such as Ewing sarcomas, Wilms' tumours, Rhabdomyosarcoma

II. **Cancer curable by chemotherapy and/or hormone therapy combined with surgery and/or radiation therapy**
     Breast cancer
     Non-small cell lung cancer (localised)
     Colon cancer
     Osteosarcoma

III. **Advanced cancer where survival can be improved by chemotherapy and/or hormone therapy**
     Breast cancer
     Non-Hodgkin's lymphoma (low-grade)
     Colon cancer
     Multiple myeloma
     Prostate cancer
     Small cell lung cancer
     Bladder cancer
     Ovarian cancer
     Rectal cancer
     Uterine cancer
     Chronic myeloid leukaemia
     Kaposi sarcoma

IV. **Advanced cancer where chemotherapy improves quality of life but with little impact on survival**
     Non-small cell lung cancer
     Cervical cancer
     Melanoma
     Oesophageal cancer
     Pancreatic cancer
     Stomach cancer
     Brain tumour
     Head and neck tumour
     Soft tissue sarcoma
     Hepatocellular cancer

V.   **Cancer that does not respond to chemotherapy**
     Renal cell cancer
     Mesothelioma (pleural cancer)
     Prostate cancer
     Uterine cancer

Clinical trials

There are four (phases in) clinical trials.

Phase I, in general, is used to test on a few select patients how high a dose of the new drug can be administered with acceptable toxic side-effects. Also referred to as a study of the right dose (a dose-finding study).

Phase II trials start once an acceptable dose has been found. The drug is then tested to ascertain its impact on the tumour and the tumour's response.

Phase III's response is compared to the response from standard chemotherapy treatment to ascertain whether the new product works better than traditional treatments.

In phase IV, the new treatment will be incorporated into main therapy for a certain cancer, alongside surgery and radiotherapy treatment.

These studies often take more than ten years to complete before the new product is made commercially available. Please note that the testing in phases I and II is done on advanced incurable cancer patients.

In order to compare the response of the tumour in these studies with each other and on an international level, certain definitions have been established (Table 2 below). 'Complete response' is defined as when, after treatment, there is no perceptible sign of the disease for at least four weeks. So a complete response rate of 50 per cent means that half of the patients tested were in 'remission' for four weeks.

The problem with this definition is that if an oncologist tells their patient that they have a 50 per cent chance of a complete response, the patient will believe that they have a 50 per cent chance of being cured, whereas the doctor knows that they have a 1-in-2 chance of the absence of all cancer symptoms for a period of four weeks. Poor communication and different expectations can be responsible for later mistrust of the doctor and a lack of trust in medicine more broadly. The patient will feel cheated and possibly do some medical shopping or attempt an unproven, often expensive, alternative 'cure'.

Please note that the definitions used for the effect of chemotherapy are based solely on the size of the tumour. They are not a measurement of the effect of chemotherapy on symptom control or on quality of life.

TABLE 2   RESPONSE TO CHEMOTHERAPY

This understanding comes from clinical trials

Complete response (CR):
  Absence of disease (at least four weeks)

Partial response (PR):
  At least 50 per cent decrease of the measured diameter of the lesions (at least four weeks)

Minor response (MR):
  Objective reduction in tumour volume (at least four weeks)

Stable disease (SD):
  No significant change in the volume of the tumour (at least four weeks)

Progressive disease (PROG):
  At least 25 per cent increase in the diameter of the lesions (at least four weeks)

Physical fitness

The patient's physical condition (performance status, PS) is an important criterion when opting for palliative chemotherapy. The most commonly used scales to measure physical condition are the Karnofsky index and the WHO or ECOG scale (see Table 3). Again these scales only reflect physical fitness and not other factors that affect quality of life.

Patients who score 40 on the Karnofsky scale survive an average of less than 50 days, while someone with a PS of 20 is likely to live only 10–20 days. Such patients are clearly not eligible for chemotherapy.

TABLE 3   SCALES FOR MEASURING PHYSICAL FITNESS
            (ECOG vs KARNOFSKY)

ECOG		Karnofsky
0	Asymptomatic	100%
1	Symptomatic; ambulatory	80–90%
2	Symptomatic; in bed <50%	60–70%
3	Symptomatic; in bed >50%	40–50%
4	Bedridden	20–30%
	Dying	10%
5	Dead	0%

Age

Although the response to chemotherapy does not usually change with age, the risk of toxicity does, particularly with regard to the decreased capacity of the blood-forming bone marrow and kidney functions. There are, of course, marked individual differences that can be explained by heredity and lifestyle. Nevertheless, doctors don't want to take risks during clinical trials, and patients over seventy seldom participate.

How long should one persevere with palliative chemotherapy?

Advanced tumours (see Table 1, p. 61) seemingly do not benefit from further treatment if there is no improvement (or stabilisation) after two cures (every three to four weeks) or after six weeks of daily or weekly treatment. At this stage it is preferable to focus on clinically improving any symptoms and quality of life. Changes in the size of the tumour are less important at this stage of the disease.

Tumours with hormonal receptors

Some tumours develop in hormonal tissues, such as breast cancer, prostate cancer and uterine cancer. Hormonal receptors have also, surprisingly, been found on other tumours: melanoma, pancreatic cancer and even lung cancer.

Long-term control can sometimes be achieved by giving hormone therapy, particularly in tumours derived from hormonally dependent tissues.

When to change chemotherapy?

When treatment (chemotherapy) results in little or no clinical improvement, it is time to consider alternative chemotherapy (second-line treatment) and then third-line chemotherapy etc. Ultimately it seems that the tumour becomes desensitised to treatment, and with each change of treatment the odds of a response dramatically decrease. For hormonally sensitive and asymptomatic breast cancer, a global response of 40 per cent is expected the first time hormones are administered, or even higher if there is no harm to internal organs. The effect of second-line treatment is already significantly less, namely 25 per cent, and only between 10 and 15 per cent by the time you reach third-line.

There is a 60 per cent response rate for first-line chemotherapy in incurable breast cancer (with 10–20 per cent complete response that can last 6–10 months). This drops to 25 per cent and less with the start of second-line treatment.

The patient's choice

Different people have different attitudes to taking risks. What is acceptable for one person is too much for another. It is therefore very difficult for doctors to decide on an acceptable level of toxicity to strike a balance between prolonging life and quality of life, another reason why mutual agreement is important. Only when the doctor is able to decide with certainty that the ultimate outcome will be negative for the patient should they refrain from treatment – if they do not do this they are indulging in futile medical treatment. It is important, however, to communicate this to the patient and their family with sensitivity in order not to lose their trust.

Palliative radiotherapy

Radiation machines

Thirty per cent of all cancer patients are cured thanks to radiotherapy. In more than 50 per cent of cases, ionising irradiation is administered with purely palliative intent.

Radiation therapy is administered via an external radiation source that emits high-energy x-rays or gamma radiation. Sometimes radioactive isotopes – radio-isotopes – are also used to administer local irradiation via a body cavity such as the vagina or a windpipe. This is called brachytherapy.

X-rays with an energy level of up to 150 kilovolts (kV) are used for superficial skin tumours or skin metastases; orthovoltage x-rays up to

300 kV penetrate to 4 cm under the skin and can still be used for palliative radiotherapy of bone metastases in the ribs or the sacrum. With the advent of cobalt machines with gamma radiation of 2.5 million volts (megavolts or MV) radiation was able to penetrate further into the human body and also reach deeply located tumours. Linear accelerators (lineacs) have now replaced the cobalt sources because they can generate even higher energetic radiation (4–25 MV). As a result, most of the energy is released internally and there is less radiation to the skin, leaving the patient 'less burnt'. The maximum energy is released at a depth that corresponds to a quarter of the energy: 6 MV gamma is released at a maximum of 1.5 cm from the skin surface. Lineacs can also produce electron beams that penetrate the skin with a penetration depth corresponding to a third of the energy of the electron beam: 9 MV electrons penetrate about 3 cm. This allows the irradiation of superficial skin lesions.

The biological impact of irradiation

High-energy irradiation has a *direct* impact in that it damages DNA molecules by the transfer of photon energy and an *indirect* impact through the ionisation of mainly water molecules inside the body cells. This creates highly toxic substances – free radicals – which in turn corrode the DNA. Most body cells have enzyme systems to repair the damage caused by irradiation. Cancer cells are less able to do this, and as a result the toxic damage accumulates in malignant tumours, while the surrounding tissue remains relatively unaffected. This difference in recovery from radiation damage is used in practice. The total lethal dose for the tumour is subdivided and administered over a number of days or weeks ('fractionation'): the healthy tissue recovers after each daily radiation session whereas the cancer cells don't recover – or at least not to the same extent. If the full dose required to kill the tumour was delivered at once, the surrounding healthy tissue would be irrevocably damaged.

Although this method spares healthy tissues, their capacity for recovery is not infinite. Irradiation also has its side-effects. The biological consequences of irradiation can be divided into early and late responses. Unlike chemotherapy, however, radiotherapy is a localised treatment. Apart from a feeling of fatigue, the side-effects are limited to the targeted area. A patient who receives radiation to their leg will not suffer from hair loss from the head.

Early reactions occur during or shortly after the irradiation itself. Depending on the irradiated area, they manifest as: an inflammation of skin and mucous membranes ('burn'), of the gastrointestinal tract (diarrhoea), a bladder infection, lung infection (pneumonitis), hair loss etc. Late effects caused by progressive damage to the irradiated tissue as a result of damage to the small blood vessels cause the irradiated tissue to die. Depending on where the radiation is administered it can result in narrowing of the oesophagus, the intestines, urethra or vagina. These effects only manifest after several months or even longer and are therefore less important in palliative treatment. There is less need for fractionation in palliative radiotherapy. The total dose is reduced because the aim is to control the symptoms not to cure the cancer.

The team of Mark De Ridder and Dirk Verellen from University Hospital Brussels recently developed a new technique that allows for very accurate targeted irradiation, thereby causing far less damage to healthy body tissue. In stereotactic radiosurgery (as it is known) the continuous positioning of the target of the irradiation is very important. In recent years this is based purely on imaging without fixation. Frameless radiosurgery is standard practice at University Hospital Brussels for treating brain metastases and provides the patient with increased reassurance.

Treating early reactions

Early reactions tend to be self-limiting and disappear after two weeks. These include skin reactions, swallowing problems, inflammation of the mucous membranes, nausea and vomiting, diarrhoea, pneumonia and bladder infections.

Palliative radiotherapy

Small doses of radiation therapy can often significantly improve the symptoms of incurable tumours. The main indications for palliative radiation therapy are compiled below. Some situations may even justify urgent irradiation.

- Local bleeding:

  Vaginal bleeding.

  Superficial bleeding from skin infiltration by tumours or metastases.

  Haemoptisis (coughing up of blood).

  Haematuria (blood puddles).

- Pain caused by tissue invasion:

  Hepatomegaly (liver enlargement from liver metastases).

  Splenomegaly (spleen enlargement from blood diseases).

  Tumours in the lower abdomen in front of the sacrum.

  Thoracic wall invasion.

- Swallowing problems:

  From intrinsic obstructions caused by oesophageal cancer or extrinsic compression from lung cancer or metastatic lymph nodes.

- Symptoms of the central nervous system:

  Double vision, epilepsy, headaches, vomiting caused by brain tumours or metastases.

- Bronchial obstruction with lung collapse as a result.

- Superior vena cava syndrome (see p.122).

- Spinal cord compression:

  By metastases (see p. 121).

- Pathologic fracture:

  Fractures caused by bone metastases will not mend. In some cases they can be fixed using orthopaedic techniques allowing the patient to once again use their limb. However, the material holding the bones together is susceptible to coming loose due to the growing metastasis. To avoid this it is best to continue radiation treatment of the area in question.

- Bone pain caused by bone metastasis:

  Even without fracture, this is very efficiently neutralised by irradiation. This is important given that this is the most common pain syndrome in cancer patients. Up to 80 per cent of the pain can be fully or partially countered in this way. The full impact manifests between one and four weeks from the start of irradiation and can last for more than half a year. For this reason irradiation is an option to consider for bone metastases even in advanced stages.

Palliative surgery

Sixty percent of all curable cancer patients can attribute their survival to surgery. This involves the complete removal of the tumour and surrounding tissue and any affected lymph nodes. Although it is fairly intrusive, patients are happy to accept it because it is the only possibility of a complete cure and survival.

Surgery is also still performed on incurable cancer patients, although highly invasive operations are usually avoided. Surgical procedures are often performed to remove the greater part of a tumour that is causing discomfort (debulking). Not all surgery is performed on the tumour itself. Sometimes the goal of the surgery is limited to resolve related problems such as placing a stoma to abrogate a bowel obstruction.

Indications for palliative surgery:

- Bleeding:

  Local bleeding such as an artery eaten away by lung cancer is often stopped by local freezing – cryotherapy – or coagulation via electrocauterisation.

- Swallowing difficulties:

  Swallowing difficulties may be caused by the narrowing of the oeso-phagus by an internal tumour or extrinsically by a mass protruding from a lung tumour or surrounding glands. Surgical dilatation of the oesophagus by placing a stent – a more or less rigid prosthesis in the form of a tube – makes it possible, in a relatively short space of time, for the patient once again to absorb food and liquids. It is also possible to place a percutaneous endoscopic gastrostomy (PEG) tube: a feeding tube is placed directly into the stomach through the abdominal wall which can then be used to get food into the patient's stomach. This is a much more comfortable option compared to the traditional gastric tube along the nasal cavity.

- Obstruction of the trachea:

  An obstruction of a main bronchus can cause severe shortness of breath, oxygen deprivation and even lung collapse. In such instances, the trachea is released using bronchoscopy and a laser or cryotherapy with or without radiotherapy. It is also possible sometimes to insert a stent.

- Pleural effusions:

  Each lung is contained within a pleural cavity which in turn is surrounded by a pleural membrane on the inside of the rib cage. Between the two pleural membranes is a vacuum which allows them to 'slide' when breathing. When malignant tumours develop in the chest, fluid can come between the two membranes causing the lung to separate from the thoracic wall and 'collapse', leaving the patient short of breath. The fluid can be drained using a 'pleural puncture'. In some patients, it comes back regularly. A more permanent solution is to inject irritants causing the two membranes to stick to each other. Talcum powder (talcage) or other products such as tetracycline can be used. Sometimes the creation of an intrapleural drain or a connection between the pleural cavity and the abdominal cavity (pleuroperitoneal shunt) can be helpful.

- Pericardial exudates or effusion:

  The heart is enclosed in a pericardial sac. A build-up of malignant fluid in this sac can quickly lead to heart failure. In some cases palliative surgical intervention is possible, but these are rather limited.

- Ascites (fluid in the abdomen):

  Obstruction of the lower hollow vein, as a result of liver metastasis for example, leads to a build-up of fluid in the abdominal cavity called ascites. Draining the fluid can offer relief both for the bowel obstruction and shortness of breath. In some cases a permanent drain is inserted.

- Obstruction of the ureter(s):

  If the ureter(s) stops functioning, urine is no longer propelled from the kidneys, and this can soon lead to kidney failure and possibly even a coma and death. Sometimes this may be the most peaceful way to die. Other times it makes sense to prevent these problems. This can be achieved by inserting a percutaneous nephrostomy: a tube is inserted directly into the renal pelvis through the patient's back connecting it directly to the skin. The urine is collected in stoma pouches. A more permanent solution is to insert ureteral stents in the bladder.

- Obstructive jaundice:

  Pancreatic cancer or metastatic glands in the region of the main bile duct block the evacuation of bile, resulting in jaundice. One possible solution is to insert a drain into the dilated bile duct. A more permanent solution would be to insert an internal stent. In non-resectable cases, a choledoco-jejunostomy can be inserted allowing the gallbladder to empty directly into the small intestine.

- Bowel obstruction:

  Obstruction of the colon is easily solved with a colostomy. Bowel obstruction caused by blockage of the small intestine is more difficult to resolve. If the blockage is localised a resection of the obstruction is worth considering, but generally the obstruction occurs in multiple places, as with metastatic ovarian tumours.

- Pathologic fractures:

  Internal reparation of long bone fractures using orthopaedic metal nails not only helps the patient become mobile quickly, it also reduces the pain. There are preventive measures that can be taken to avoid pathological fractures and the subsequent misery. These are usually taken when the metastatic bone decalcification is more than 2.5 cm with deterioration of the periosteum or cortex.

- Metastases:

  Single brain metastases can be surgically removed, thereby significantly improving the patient's quality of life. It may even prolong the patient's life for a few months if treatment is continued. Surgery can also be considered for certain lung metastases.

Palliative surgery can so often bring relief to incurable patients. As always, the expected result needs to be weighed up against the potential mortality rate.

Other incurable diseases

Not only incurable cancer patients are eligible for (active) treatment. Nowadays there are ways of treating other incurable diseases by the proper application of the available medical high technology, thus improving the quality of and even prolonging patients' lives.

In fact, incurable diseases are responsible for the vast majority of healthcare. Most illnesses are (still) incurable although they can usually be treated reasonably well with long-lasting effect. Examples are: chronic pulmonary disease, heart failure, kidney failure, HIV/AIDS, amyotrophic lateral sclerosis (ALS) (also known as motor neurone disease, or MND), multiple sclerosis, Parkinson's disease, diabetes, osteoarthritis, arteriosclerosis, chronic hepatitis, osteoporosis, Crohn's disease, Alzheimer's and non-congenital brain conditions such as the effects of a coma after a traffic accident etc.

Among all these incurable disorders there are also serious, life-threatening diseases that, despite active treatment, have an increasing effect on the patient and limit their life expectancy. In addition, these non-oncological but nevertheless seriously ill non-cancer patients often experience similar symptoms to those experienced by seriously ill cancer patients, especially during the final stages. Then again, the dying process of these patients differs from cancer patients in that terminal cancer patients usually go downhill rapidly, whereas the deterioration in other serious diseases usually takes longer and is interspersed with acute outbreaks that can be treated reasonably well in the hospital or in a palliative care unit.

Optimal active treatment is best achieved when the organ specialist of the given condition, for example the cardiologist, consults with the palliative doctor or palliative team.

Some of these diseases and their specific active treatment are briefly explained here, and for those that are not covered, such as dementia, many excellent books are available. *Simultaneous* support for medical complaints and symptoms (for example shortness of breath and confusion) together with psychosocial and spiritual care – palliative care through and through – is covered in Chapters 7–10.

The final stage of these diseases is briefly outlined, as much less is known about them than the terminal stage of cancer.

Chronic pulmonary disease

Chronic pulmonary disease (for example chronic bronchitis or emphysema) is often caused by continual inhalation of fine dust, as with smoking, working in a dusty environment without protection for the respiratory tract etc. Pulmonary disease often develops gradually with periods of unbearable shortness of breath which usually requires urgent hospitalisation. The main symptoms during the terminal phase include shortness of breath, coughing, fever, haemoptysis, rasping, noisy breathing and pain in the chest region. These symptoms are very similar to those of a terminal lung-cancer patient.

Shortness of breath and coughing often have a negative impact on the patient's quality of life. Respiratory distress can lead to reduced food intake and constipation due to the extra effort required. Acute shortness of breath can cause anxiety and sometimes even induce panic.

Chronic lack of oxygen in the blood (hypoxemia) should be avoided as far as possible. The degree of saturation of oxygen in the blood should be more than 90 per cent – if this is not the case, the heart is overworked and this could lead to secondary heart failure (cor pulmonale). Shortness of breath can be countered with morphine and benzodiazepines (see p. 104, Annex, p. 223). In cases where the patient is completely exhausted, a (short) sedation (artificial sleep) may even be considered.

Physiotherapy can help improve the patient's breathing technique: teaching them how to suppress the coughing reflex, remove the mucous reflux caused, for example, by cystic fibrosis. See p. 117 for additional methods to combat coughing.

Active treatment

The treatment of chronic pulmonary disease is somewhat limited. Puffers (bronchodilators) with anticholinergics and/or beta-agonists should be used for as long as possible to keep the airway open. Trial therapy using corticoids can be considered for the same reason.

Anti-inflammatories and antibiotics are used to reduce the lung damage caused by chronic infection.

Chronic heart failure

All advanced cardiovascular diseases (especially damage to the coronary arteries and high blood pressure) lead to chronic heart failure unless the patient suddenly dies (from a heart attack or a fatal arrhythmia). Heart failure manifests itself by a malfunction of the heart's pump function. This then sets off a series of complications in the metabolism, blood vessels, hormones and kidney functions.

Heart diseases often progress at unpredictable rates, which means they are difficult to treat and require recurrent hospitalisation. The severity of cardiac decompensation is frequently underestimated by many patients and their friends and family; neither are there any reliable criteria with which doctors can predict imminent death. In addition, the final stage of heart failure is more deadly than many cancers: 40 per cent die within the year and only 20 per cent live longer than five years. The main symptoms in this stage are: oedemas (especially in the legs) causing shortness of breath, coughing and fatigue, nausea, anorexia, weight loss and cachexia (see p. 98), pain (also caused by swelling of the liver), constipation, reduced mobility, insomnia, confusion, anaemia, a drop in blood pressure when standing up quickly, anxiety and depression.

Ensuring that these symptoms receive the best possible treatment will help keep the number of hospital admissions down (see Chapter 7). It is particularly important to pay special attention to oedemas: these grow due to retention of fluid in tissues because the heart's pump function is weaker. They can be treated with diuretics such as furosemide (Lasix®), combined with a reduction in salt and fluid intake (maximum of 1500–2000 ml per day) as well as placing a pillow under the legs. Morphine preparations, benzodiazepines and dissolving glyceryl tri-nitrate tablets under the tongue are used to combat shortness of breath, and nonsteroidal anti-inflammatory products such as Voltaren® and corticoids are avoided when trying to reduce pain, as they lead to greater fluid retention.

Dietary advice is a valuable consideration, and even moderate alcohol consumption can help increase the appetite and reduce anxiety.

The impact of chronic cardiac decompensation should not be underestimated on a physical, psychological and social level. The New York Heart Association has developed a functional classification system to help physicians to determine the best course of therapy.

TABLE 4   NEW YORK HEART ASSOCIATION SYSTEM FOR
            THE CLASSIFICATION OF CHRONIC CARDIAC
            DECOMPENSATION SYMPTOMS

Class	Symptoms
I	Cardiac malaise with limited shortness of breath
II	Comfortable at rest but respiratory distress during daily activities
III	Respiratory distress during any activity resulting in limited physical functionality
IV	Respiratory distress at rest

Active treatment

There is limited treatment available for heart failure, and what little there is is based on digitalis preparations to support the heart muscle in conjunction with substances to lower the blood pressure, such as angiotensin converting enzyme (ACE) inhibitors and angiotensin receptor blocking agents.

Chronic renal (kidney) failure

Chronic kidney failure occurs when the kidney's filter function stops working properly (less than 10 ml per minute). The only ways to overcome the problem are through kidney dialysis or a kidney transplant. Between 10 and 20 per cent of patients with chronic kidney failure die every year. Most kidney patients die from the associated diseases that are the cause of the kidney failure, particularly cardiovascular diseases. Another frequent cause of kidney failure is diabetes, which in itself is also a major health problem.

A significant number of patients in the course of dialysis ask to stop or even not to start in the first place. These decisions not to treat the condition require a thorough ethical consultation (see p. 139). Patients who do not undergo dialysis (or who stop) survive for an average of ten days, during which time they will require intensive palliative care.

Many symptoms are caused by the dialysis itself: itching, 'restless legs', cramps, drowsiness, low blood pressure and nausea. In addition, about half of all dialysis patients complain of (nerve) pain. When morphine is prescribed it is important also to consider any toxic metabolites produced by the affected kidney function that are no longer evacuated in the urine and so continue to circulate in the body. It may be better to use a 'morphine-like' painkiller with no toxic waste (see pp. 89 and 217).

AIDS

The human immunodeficiency virus (HIV) infection after a few years develops into acquired immunodeficiency syndrome (AIDS) with a fatal prognosis. The HIV virus affects the CD4 protein in the immune system's white blood cells (T4-cells) leaving the patient highly susceptible to infection (once their CD4 count drops to less than 200/microlitre). These infections are often caused by opportunistic micro-organisms such as bacteria, viruses, fungi and single-celled protozoa (for example tuberculosis, pneumocystis carinii pneumonia, cryptococcal meningitis, cytomegalovirus infection, toxoplasmosis, herpes zoster). For the same reason, AIDS patients are also more susceptible to certain malignant tumours such as Kaposi's sarcoma and brain lymphoma.

The HIV virus also infects other body tissues, resulting in chronic diarrhoea and incontinence, weight loss, cachexia and fatigue, muscle and joint pain, painful deterioration of the nerves (neuropathy), oedemas, respiratory distress and coughing, nausea, convulsions, confusion and progressive dementia, fever, itching, ulcerations at the mucous membranes of the mouth and the genitals, visual impairment, and damage to the blood cells, with anaemia and coagulation problems. Anxiety attacks, periods of depression and psychological problems complete the clinical picture.

AIDS is unpredictable in the way it develops, with periods of acute pain during which the physical condition of the patient deteriorates dramatically. Palliative care is therefore needed long before the patient enters the terminal phase. Even during the 'quiet' phase of the disease, when the virus content ('viral load') in the blood is controlled by medication, HIV patients are often stigmatised and socially isolated, and as a result are not always committed to ensuring good medical care and may even stop their intensive treatment.

Recently there has been a worrying increase in the number of HIV infections. This may be explained by unprotected sex due to false reassurances that life-saving (but still not curative) medication is available.

Active treatment

Antivirus products such as reverse transcriptase and protease inhibitors as well as 'highly active antiretroviral therapy' or HAART are used in the active treatment of AIDS. Since its introduction, HAART has been able to help patients who are already at an advanced stage to improve rapidly (the 'Lazarus syndrome') and keep the AIDS patients under control for long periods. HAART treatment is normally started when the CD4 count drops below 200/microlitre. Other treatments include:

- treatment of infections with antibiotics etc.;
- treatment of secondary cancers such as Kaposi's sarcoma by means of palliative chemotherapy and radiotherapy.

Amyotrophic lateral sclerosis (ALS)

ALS is an attack from an unknown source on the nerve cells responsible for muscle movement (the motor neurons). In the UK it is known as motor neurone disease. After a period of progressive weakness, paralysis and other symptoms, the patient dies after an average or three to four years. Palliative care therefore begins as soon as the patient has been diagnosed.

The symptoms stem from the nerve damage: muscle weakness, spasticity and cramps, difficulty swallowing, speech difficulties, breathlessness with attacks of 'choking' and extreme fear, thickened mucus (due to reduced fluid intake and diminished ability to cough), muscle and bone pain, inappropriate 'laughing and weeping', constipation and insomnia. All these problems require a multidisciplinary approach: physiotherapy to preserve muscle function as long as possible, speech therapy and dietary advice for swallowing and speech difficulties, and discussion of the pros and cons of inserting a stomach tube and/or assisted ventilation etc.

Ninety per cent of ALS patients die in their sleep.

Active treatment

- Riluzole is the only drug that has a limited positive effect, and can prolong the patient's life for about three months.
- Stomach probe and/or assisted ventilation.

A special group: incurably sick children

The death of a child is one of the greatest tragedies that can happen to a family. Infant mortality in newborn babies used not to be an exception, but thanks to modern medicine (in the Western industrialised world at least) it is now prevented more often than not. Fortunately, also, fatal diseases such as cancer are very rare in children. About a hundred thousand people in Belgium die every year, of whom fewer than a thousand are under 18 years of age, although this is little consolation to parents who have lost a child. I have therefore included this short section on the principles of active treatment of incurably sick minors.

Fortunately there are now effective active treatments for many conditions such as cancer, which accounts for 40 per cent of children's deaths. Cancer used to have a mortality rate of more than 50 per cent among children (and adults) but now, thanks to new developments in therapy, well over 50 per cent of children with cancer survive (and sometimes up to 80 per cent). Very intense active and sometimes aggressive treatment with the potential to cure is therefore frequently applied for extended periods. This makes any transition to 'palliation' much more difficult. Another consequence is that the child and their parents develop a strong bond with the attendant medical team. These two factors combined can result in the parents being less amenable to a 'strange' palliative care team and preferring to stick with the original team. Several years ago, Professor Yves Benoit, paediatric oncologist at University Hospital Ghent, therefore founded the successful Koester project with support from Kom op tegen Kanker. Specially trained nurses from the Paediatric Oncology unit at University Hospital Ghent visit advanced cancer patients in their homes. This gives the patients and their parents a feeling of continuity of care from a trusted source. The patient can also then stay at home for as long as possible. The same philosophy is followed by other large paediatric oncology centres such as University Hospital Leuven. The Belgian legislation of 5 March 2009 also recognises the financing of palliative home-care teams for children.

Most children with life-shortening conditions would prefer to be cared for at home.

They can be divided into four categories:

- curable diseases where the treatment has failed;
- diseases that lead to premature death but where intensive life-prolonging treatment is combined with a good quality of life;
- progressive disorders which are treated with palliative care from the beginning and may last for several years;
- incurable but not progressive disorders which are highly susceptible to complications and are likely to cause premature death.

Sick children are special because they are totally dependent on adults not only for their care and protection but also when taking (ethical) decisions. The older they get the more independent they become and the more able to look after themselves and make their own decisions. The natural instinct to want to protect a seriously ill child can therefore enter into conflict with the needs of the growing child, particularly if the sickness drags on for years. Moreover, long-term sick children are often more mentally mature than the average adolescent partygoer. Parents and healthcare professionals are therefore constantly having to find the right balance. Children generally know more than they are given credit for, and so it is best to keep them informed as much as possible and involved in decision-making without losing sight of the value of short-term projects, such as a visit to Disneyland.

The same applies to grandparents and siblings, the latter frequently being forgotten or given less attention, and thus referred to as 'shadow children' – this can lead to serious psychological problems.

In order to support such families, a pioneer in palliative care, Colette Raymakers, opened, in the presence of Minister Jo Vandeurzen among others, the first respite (specialist care) home in a former monastery in De Panne on 30 June 2010. It was named Villa Rozerood (Red Rose Villa) and acts as a pleasant refuge for incurable children, their parents and the shadow children.

Pain and symptom control in children is no different from that for adults. The only difference is the quantity of medication. Newborns have a relatively higher percentage of body fluid and a slower discharge of urine, and should therefore be given smaller doses than adults. Young children, older than six months, are able to break down certain medication faster than adults and so require relatively more morphine.

Conclusion

The above-mentioned serious incurable diseases – in adults and children – are not the only diseases to require palliative care. Other chronic diseases and their environments are rightly being recognised as needing palliative care: psychiatric patients, patients with dementia, patients with Parkinson's disease, patients with multiple sclerosis and patients with an acquired brain injury (ABI). These patients are just as much in need of palliative (supportive) care to complement their active treatment as are patients who have reached the terminal phase of their disease (see Chapters 7–10).

7 Pain and symptom control

Someone who is continually vomiting has little concern for metaphysical considerations.

Introduction

One important aspect that is often forgotten during active treatment to extend a patient's life (such as chemotherapy or radiotherapy) is the impact on their quality of life. Doctors, too often, focus on the post-treatment results and pay little heed to the patient's suffering. Pain reduction after bone metastasis radiation, for example, takes several weeks to kick in and the patient therefore requires early pain-relief medication as well as psychological support for the realisation that their cancer has spread. The same applies to the active treatment of other incurable diseases: attention to physical discomfort and psychological problems *during* treatment for heart failure, for example, or while giving drug treatment to a patient with AIDS.

Every attempt should of course be made to restrict the side-effects of active treatment. It cannot be stressed too highly that awareness of and attention to signs and symptoms must not be limited to the terminal phase of treatment. Palliative care should not be restricted to terminal care, but should support the active treatment of incurable diseases. This *supportive* care must be an indispensable element of the treatment of incurable patients from the point of diagnosis. Palliative care therefore consists of supportive care and terminal care (including bereavement care). The correct attitude and basic empathy are crucial.

After consultation the doctor should quickly be able to assess what the patient considers to be important for their quality of life. Direct questions such as 'what is the biggest burden for you at the moment?' can help ascertain and thus address the most urgent complaints. There is no symptom hierarchy. One patient may be driven to distraction by generalised itching whereas another may find the fear of death harder to bear. In principle, the patient is always right. Even if their complaints are 'imaginary' they are no less real.

If the healthcare professional is able to relieve the primary complaint (even partially) it helps to gain the patient's trust in treating other symptoms. In all cases, it is important to give priority to the complaint that troubles the patient the most, and not what the healthcare professional thinks is most urgent. Untreated anaemia seems very important but does not cause the patient any distress, whereas an inflamed oral mucosa can cause severe discomfort.

Similarly, during the curative phase, the healthcare professionals strive to combat the cause as much as possible. Vomiting can just as easily be caused by brain metastases as a stomach irritation, although the treatment is obviously different. It often happens that the cause of a particular complaint is not easy to diagnose (chronic nausea for example). In such instances the trial-and-error method is used to find the most effective solution. Patients are generally happy with this approach provided they are kept informed, for example 'Give me a few days to solve the problem, because I want to help you in the best way possible.' Attention to detail is fundamental, for example a patient who indicates that their nausea is worse when lying on their back (because of regurgitation of stomach fluids). Observation can also help to find a solution. Not all short-term complaints necessarily need to be treated.

In curative medicine treatment stops once the patient is cured. Antibiotics are stopped once the pneumonia has cleared up. In serious incurable diseases, however, the treatment continues. There is a constant search for the right cure for the right complaint at the right time. An anti-vomiting medicine can lose its effectiveness after a while, and then a few months later it appears to work again after a period during which other alternatives were used successfully.

When changing medication, it is normal to change one medicine at a time so as to be able to ascertain which medicine helped to combat the symptoms or caused side-effects.

In cases of serious complaints such as excruciating pain it is important to be available for the patient. Regular evaluations are carried out and further treatment is based on the findings. Allowing a patient to contact their physician by phone helps to reassure the patient as well as their family and friends; it helps to build trust.

It is not helpful, however, to relieve the patient of all of their complaints only to replace them with more side-effects as a result. The level of relief must be determined by the patient. For example, some would rather suffer a certain degree of pain rather than have their mental faculties impaired. They want to be able to read the newspaper and watch television, whereas others prefer complete pain relief and so accept the drowsiness and reduced concentration as part of the package.

With less coherent patients it is appropriate to actively ask questions about their condition: 'Are you in pain?', 'What do think about most?', 'Are you sleeping well at night?', 'How's your appetite?' These simple questions can reveal underestimated symptoms.

It is important also for the healthcare professional always to appear relaxed. Even when in a hurry their body language should give the opposite impression. Sitting on a chair or the edge of the bed lowers the patient's aversion (intimidation) to discussing problems. In addition, being in a sitting position establishes horizontal eye contact so that no-one is 'looking down' at the other. Being mindful of these details helps the patients feel more at ease. They are fundamental when dealing with patients with serious problems who have lost their autonomy and self-sufficiency. The feeling of being able to maintain a certain level of control and to be seen as 'whole' improves their self-image and self-esteem.

Dealing with terminally ill people is a balance between sufficient empathy and the expert application of knowledge and skills. On the one hand it implies being critical of the futility of certain routine actions and examinations, such as measuring blood pressure, taking the temperature or conducting radiography checks. If a particular test result leads to no change in strategy or outcome there is no sense, strictly speaking, in conducting the examination. On the other hand, patients are quick to sense that something is not right when certain examinations are stopped. It is therefore very important to continue with physical examinations, not necessarily to discover a pressure ulcer wound, for example, but because it reassures patients that they are, as a whole, important to the healthcare professional.

Finally, one should not be confined to the arsenal of medicines or classic nursing techniques. It is important to listen to what the patient thinks will help to alleviate their discomfort: a massage, a bath with ethereal oils, relaxing music, smoking a cigarette and drinking a glass of wine or placing the sickbed near a window with a view. All it takes is a bit of empathy, awareness and creativity (see 'Attention to detail', p.119), and hence the importance of the complementary role fulfilled by volunteers.

Interestingly, regardless of the textbook or publication consulted (a recent publication or one dating back ten years), the main symptoms remain the same.

The most common symptoms are:

- pain;
- fear;
- anorexia, cachexia;
- shortness of breath;
- constipation;
- delirium;
- depression;
- nausea and vomiting.

Less common symptoms are:

- ascites;
- bladder spasms and bladder irritation;
- diarrhoea;
- bowel obstruction;
- hiccups;

- coughing;
- itching;
- oedemas;
- pleural effusions.

We will discuss these problems in more depth. Readers who are interested in (technical) details of some treatments can refer to the Annex (see p. 207).

Pain

On 11 October 2004, the first Global Day Against Pain was organised to underline the extent of the problem. One fifth of the world's population suffers from moderate to severe chronic pain, with one third no longer able to function normally while carrying out every day domestic activities, exercising, sleeping, at social functions, driving, hiking and engaging in sexual activities. Almost one in four Europeans suffers from chronic pain.

Finding ways to relieve pain clearly illustrates the need to approach patients as a whole. Dame Cicely Saunders first introduced the concept of 'total pain'. All symptoms are affected by many different factors. In order to treat a complaint optimally it is important to take all of these factors into account.

The International Association for the Study of Pain (IASP) issued this definition of pain (1979): 'Pain is an unpleasant sensory and emotional experience, which is associated with actual or potential tissue damage or described in terms of damage.' Pain is thus experienced by the whole person and is more than just physical discomfort. Pain is a multidimensional phenomenon that requires care for the whole person; total care.

Severe chronic pain is mainly treated with medication, but it is important also to consider underlying emotional and psychosocial factors as well as non-drug pain management such as physiotherapy, radiotherapy, chemotherapy or surgical intervention.

The WHO in Geneva published a booklet in 1986, with a re-issue in 1996, of almost eighty pages describing ways of treating cancer pain. It has been translated into most world languages but somehow failed to reach healthcare professionals who needed it most. Of course the basic rules for treating cancer pain described below also apply to all other forms of chronic pain. For more technical details about pain therapy, see the Annex, p. 208.

Cancer pain and other chronic pain can be very effectively countered

One in four people dies of cancer, and with the ageing population it will soon be one in three. Cancer pain is present in 50 per cent of the patients in the early stages of the diagnosis and 75 per cent of patients in the advanced stages. Pain in most cancer patients is undertreated because of lack of knowledge among healthcare professionals.

And yet, up to 90 per cent of these painful symptoms can be effectively countered or at least reduced to a level where they no longer dominate everything: patients can once again think about things other than pain. Moreover, pain control is very easily achieved by the regular ingestion of certain medicines.

Principles of pain management by drugs

Cancer pain is mainly caused by the spread of the tumour itself, such as: by metastases of the bone structure, nerve compression, organ deterioration or failure, or spreading to the lymph nodes. To a lesser extent the pain is caused by cancer therapy, namely pain following surgical interventions, chemotherapy or radiotherapy.

The booklet published by the WHO emphasises a very important principle: administer the *correct dose* of the *right medicine, orally, at the right time.*

Which is the right medicine?

It is better to have in-depth knowledge of the effect and side-effects of a handful of drugs than to have superficial knowledge about many products.

Orally

Pain relief for chronic pain should preferably be administered through the mouth (orally). The pain control thus obtained is as effective as from drugs administered via an injection into a vein or into muscle. The only difference is that sometimes slightly higher doses need to be administered in order to compensate for the *first pass* effect in the liver, namely the breaking down of the drug by the liver after passing through the stomach. In addition, pain relief via oral medication takes longer to have an effect. Given that painkillers in chronic cases are administered at very strict intervals, the difference between oral and intravenous ingestion will only be noticeable when first administered.

The main argument for administering painkillers orally is quality of life. This way, the patient remains mobile and independent as well as being able to learn to adjust the daily dose themselves. And on top of that, a visit to the hospital is avoided.

The right time

Many widely used painkillers only work for a few hours. It would clearly be illogical to administer a drug which lasts four hours every eight hours. Chronic pain is present permanently and often increases as the disease evolves. Statements often heard from healthcare professionals such as 'give painkillers if the patient asks' or 'only give painkillers when necessary' do not apply here. Such treatment would only create a vicious cycle of pain-free periods followed by periods of chronic pain. Patients then become more difficult to treat and lose confidence in the ability of the painkillers to relieve pain, and the healthcare professional is then more likely to administer a stronger painkiller. If the exact duration of the drug's effectiveness is not known, it can be found on the package leaflet.

The correct dose

It is important to administer the correct dose of any product. Most painkillers not derived from morphine have a maximum dosage, a so-called ceiling effect: after a certain stage, there is no point in increasing the dose any further as it will not deliver better pain relief but may well increase the side-effects. In such cases a more powerful medicine is required.

A common mistake in good pain control is to want to reduce the morphine dose. Most chronic diseases are progressive; the pain will worsen rather than diminish. This requires the amount of medication to be adjusted, usually increased. If it is possible to achieve pain control without drugs, by irradiation of painful bone metastases for example, then it will be possible to reduce the dose of painkillers.

To help gain worldwide acceptance of the basics of pain management the WHO has introduced the concept of the 'pain ladder'.

The pain ladder

The pain ladder is a very practical tool in helping select the correct analgesic. It contains three steps and is limited to standard medication. The prototypes that belong to each level respectively are Aspirin®, codeine and morphine. Alternatives exist for each of these products.

Step 1: weak non-morphine-like products

A patient with limited pain is the first step and requires non-morphine-like substances. Prototypes are Dafalgan®, Aspirin® or any other NSAID (non-steroidal anti-inflammatory drug) such as Indocid®, Brufen®, Voltaren®, Apranax® and Celebrex®.

If these products are administered correctly – the right dose at the right time – and the patient continues to feel pain, it is necessary to move to step 2 of the ladder and start with morphine preparations. Since step 1 medicines work differently to morphine-like products one should continue to administer these products during step 2 and step 3.

Step 2: weak morphine-like products

The prototype is codeine. Alternatives are Codicontin®, tramadol, Contramal® and Dolzam®.

Once these painkillers are no longer sufficient to relieve the pain, the patient moves to the third and final step of the analgesics ladder; strong morphine-like products with or without products from step 1. There is no point in combining weak morphine-like products (step 2) with strong opioids. Codeine and morphine will not be administered together as they both have the same mode of action.

Step 3: strong morphine-like products

When weak analgesics no longer relieve the pain, it is time to administer morphine. Morphine can be consumed in syrup or pill form (MS Direct®, MS Contin®), drops or solution (Oramorph®). Alternatives to morphine are Palladone®, Oxycontin® and Mephenon® (methadone). Durogesic® or Transtec® patches can also be used.

FIGURE 2   THE PAIN LADDER

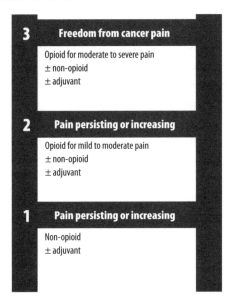

Why does morphine have such a bad reputation?

Morphine is found in opium, which is the dried sap obtained from the opium poppy (*papaver somniferum*). Its calming, euphoria-inducing, sleep-inducing and analgesic properties have been known since thousands of years before Christ. The plant was used for various purposes, primarily in the Far East, but also in the Mediterranean, and famous Greeks such as Homer, Hippocrates and Aristotle wrote about its properties. The word itself comes from the Greek and means sap, and by extension papaver sap.

Opium was introduced into China by Arab traders around the year 400. Thereafter people began to cultivate it in China, India and Indonesia. As a result of the Inquisition, opium was taboo in Europe between the twelfth and fifteenth centuries: merchandise from the East was regarded as being of the devil. At the end of the fifteenth century, exotic products such as opium were again introduced into Europe by Vasco da Gama from India and by the British from China. Despite Paracelsus, around 1500, and Thomas Sydenham in the seventeenth century introducing opium as medicine, it was mostly used in the Middle East for recreational purposes, often mixed with tobacco in a Turkish water pipe. By the end of the seventeenth century opium-smoking became a real trend for the Dutch in the Philippines and South China. The Chinese emperor Yung Cheng tried to contain the addictive habit by introducing smoking salons ('opium kits') and banning the sale of opium. Nevertheless, the British continued to import massive amounts of opium through the East India Company. This led to two Opium Wars between China and Great Britain in the nineteenth century, culminating in Hong Kong being handed over to the British and the legalisation of the opium trade. The use of opium also took hold in Europe and was praised by famous figures such as John Keats, Guillaume Apollinaire and Jules Verne.

In 1803 the German, Friedrich Sertürner, extracted morphine by dissolving opium in acid and neutralising it with ammonia. The product was then marketed by the company Merck. Then, in 1843, the Scotsman Alexander Wood suggested that injecting morphine into a vein made the effects three times stronger. In 1874, an Englishman, Alder Wright, synthesised heroin by cooking morphine on a stove. Heroin, or diamorphine as it is also known, is produced when two morphine molecules come together.

Until around 1900, the recreational use of opium was considered too addictive and the British Opium Act (1878) proposed an end to the sale of opium in China and India. In 1909, it became illegal to import opium into the United States. This was the beginning of strict regulations governing the trade in opiates. Opium became illegal and the 'narcotics business' was conducted mainly by the mafia.

This colourful history explains why the use of opium derivatives such as morphine still evokes so much resistance. Even for purely medical use such as pain relief, the deeply ingrained prejudices are still present, and too many doctors hesitate to prescribe enough morphine. This aversion is present also among pharmacists. This causes unnecessary concern for patients suffering from chronic pain. They perceive this resistance as the ultimate proof that their prognosis is very bad. The myths surrounding morphine persist, and as a result many chronic pain problems are undertreated.

What are opiates?

All products derived from natural opium are called opiates. They come from the poppy plant. Well-known opiates are morphine, codeine, and papaverine.

What are opioids?

Opioids are not restricted to morphine, codeine and papaverine but also include all other natural or (semi-)synthetic substances whose effects are mediated by specific receptors in the central and peripheral nervous system and whose activity can be blocked by the antagonist naloxone. All opiates are opioids, but the reverse does not apply. The synthetic product methadone is an opioid but not an opiate. Morphine is an opiate and an opioid.

What are narcotics?

The term is derived from the Greek 'narke', meaning 'numb'. It is used to describe morphine-like products in the drug environment. Given its pejorative connotation it is best avoided when dealing with pain relief.

What are receptors?

'Receptors' is the name given to molecules in the cell (membrane) that act as specific binding sites for certain substances, for example μ-receptors for opioids, α- and β-receptors for adrenalin, the receptors for acetylcholine and for different hormones. When these substances attach themselves to the receptor molecule, the cell responds, with the result that certain cellular functions are enhanced or inhibited. There are at least three types of opioid receptors: morphine receptor μ (mu), the κ (kappa) receptor and the enkephalin receptor δ (delta). These receptors are located in the brain, spinal cord and peripheral nerve endings.

Each receptor type responds slightly differently. In addition, certain opioids attach themselves to more than one receptor with varying affinity. This explains why the above-mentioned side-effects of certain opioids are more pronounced than those of a different opioid. It also explains why it is useful to rotate opioids (see p. 88).

The NMDA receptor (N-methyl D-aspartate) located in the central nervous system also has a modulating effect on pain. There are substances that hinder the presynaptic re-uptake of serotonin and norepinephrine between nerve cells, such as the antidepressants known as SSRIs (selective serotonin reuptake inhibitors). The effect is to reduce pain stimuli caused by direct damage to the nerve itself. This is also referred to as neuropathic pain.

Response to activating the μ-, κ- and δ-receptors:

μ   analgesia, respiratory depression, miosis (small pupils), euphoria, decreased gastrointestinal movement;

κ   analgesia, dysphoria, psychomimetic effects such as hallucinations, miosis, respiratory depression

δ   analgesia, no additional side-effects.

> **Why do we have morphine receptors?**
>
> Several small proteins (peptides) with morphine-like properties have been found in the human body: endorphins (μ-receptor), dynorfins (κ-receptor) and enkephalins (δ-receptor).
>
> The opioid peptides are therefore neurotransmitters and belong to a complicated blocking signal system. They block, among others, incoming pain signals. They are believed to have played an important role in the fight-and-flight reaction during the evolution of mammals, allowing them to survive under extreme stress. In the case of soldiers with severed limbs who continue fighting or run away, the pain is made bearable thanks to the activation of endorphins. Jogging releases endogenous morphines which can explain why people become 'addicted' to jogging. The analgesic effect of acupuncture might also be based on the release of endorphins.

There is also talk of a fourth step, the fitting of an epidural catheter through which painkillers are injected into the patient's spinal fluid. The indications for such an application are, in practice, limited.

Unfortunately, there are many misconceptions and myths surrounding morphine.

Myths about morphine

As a result of the many ingrained prejudices and misconceptions about morphine, it is under-prescribed, leaving too many patients to endure horrific pain.

What are the most common myths?

Addiction

Morphine leads to addiction. Enough studies on patients with severe chronic pain have been done to show the contrary. These patients do not become addicted or psychologically dependent. Some even spontaneously stop taking morphine: they forget to take their pill every now and then and they find their pain is bearable, or if the pain is controlled in some other way, such as irradiation of painful bone metastases.

Tolerance

Many healthcare professionals believe that morphine use leads to tolerance. They believe that sustained use of morphine would mean that it would no longer be effective at the moment when it is most needed. This misconception is based on findings in recreational drug users. It is true that after a while they have to use more and more morphine or heroin to get the same kick. This has nothing to do with pain medication. In cancer patients, the need to increase the morphine dose is directly related to the increase in pain as the disease progresses.

Respiratory depression

In patients suffering with chronic pain there is no risk of respiratory depression from morphine. This mistaken belief comes from a study on post-operative pain in the 1960s. Patients were administered a standard dose of morphine after surgery. In addition, the patients were recovering from a chloroform anaesthetic which can compromise breathing. For some, the morphine dose proved to be too high, which exacerbated any breathing difficulty that the patient was experiencing.

These conditions cannot be compared to problems caused by chronic pain. The morphine dose is regularly adjusted according to pain levels. Pain is one of the most powerful stimuli of the respiratory centre and in fact morphine is sometimes prescribed to relieve shortness of breath.

Morphine turns patients into zombies

Patients on morphine supposedly walk around like zombies or indeed the *living dead*. This line of thought is well illustrated by a statement made by a doctor: 'I try to postpone morphine treatment for as long as possible and preferably leave it until the end. I'm most satisfied if the first dose of morphine also turns out to be the last.' This reasoning is based on reports of people who have been given an overdose of morphine, or pain-free drug abusers.

When morphine is prescribed, death is imminent

Many associate the use of morphine with an imminent death. Nevertheless there is ample evidence that the opposite is true. A pain-free patient who sleeps better, has a bigger appetite and gets out of bed more as a result of morphine will be less susceptible to pneumonia, for example, which has fatal consequences.

Morphine is also administered to patients with severe pain caused by advanced debilitating arthritis, a non-life-threatening disease.

Morphine increases suicide rates

Fears that patients on morphine are likely to commit suicide are unjustified. There is sufficient evidence to show that the incidence of suicide among cancer patients is not significantly higher than in healthy people.

Adjuvants or additives

Painkillers can be supported on each step of the ladder by so-called adjunctive medication. These 'additives' either improve the effect of the painkillers (and are therefore also known as co-analgesics) or they reduce their side-effects, for example laxatives, anti-vomiting pills and psycho-stimulants.

The use of co-analgesics was introduced because certain chronic pain syndromes cannot be properly controlled by morphine. An example of partially morphine-resistant pain is soft tissue pain, such as muscle pain, or increased pressure in the skull caused by brain metastases. Muscle spasm and nerve damage (neuropathic pain) are inadequately controlled by morphine. Nerve pain manifests itself as a superficial burning sensation, accompanied by 'shooting' pain. There may also be a deep, dull component. Damage to the autonomic nervous system manifests itself initially as vasodilation – red, swollen and 'burning' skin – and subsequently transpiration.

The effects and side-effects of co-analgesics are difficult be predict because they vary significantly. For this reason it is appropriate to try them one after the other. And, as always, the patient should be informed of what is happening in order to earn and maintain their trust.

Certain co-analgesics have a specific influence on the central nervous system and hence are known as psychotropic additives. The effects of these psychotropic drugs, such as anti-depressants, can be useful in treating the above-mentioned concept of 'total pain', but have nothing to do with the medicamentous approach to cortical influences such as depression.

Fear

Anxiety in patients with (advanced) cancer or other serious conditions such as AIDS is frequently caused by the diagnosis itself: the doomsday picture of untreatable pain and other symptoms, the side-effects of the treatment, the progressive loss of autonomy and the culmination in death. This fear is often reinforced by previous experiences of patients with 'similar' conditions.

In addition, many patients fear that their illness will become a burden for their friends and family. The anticipative realisation of loss of control and independence can be unbearable.

Fear can fluctuate in intensity while being examined or undergoing procedures and waiting for the results.

Anxiety can be triggered by organ deterioration: pain, oxygen deprivation, delirium (see p. 106).

In addition, fear can often be masked by denial, insomnia, nightmares and attention-seeking behaviour.

And finally, fear and anxiety can be triggered by having to give up alcohol, tobacco, opioids or benzodiazepines. Conversely, it can be caused by certain medications which provoke akathisia: internal unrest and fear, nervous movements, jumping from one foot to the other and the inability to sit or stand still. This occurs with certain neuroleptics such as metoclopramide and haloperidol (Haldol®). Fortunately these symptoms can easily be eliminated by the patient processing the medication and the doctor prescribing a benzodiazepine.

Assessing the level of anxiety

The patient should be asked about:
- previous experiences with anxiety and coping strategies;
- which physical complaints cause anxiety;
- what occupies their mind;
- their opinions about their health and prognosis.

The physical and psychological signs of anxiety manifest as:
- becoming sweaty, pale or glowing red;
- hypertension, palpitations, accelerated breathing, diarrhoea, stomach upset;
- irritation;
- being worried, trembling, strained, unable to focus;
- instability, hyper-alertness, overattentiveness.

In addition, there may be changes to the patient's behaviour such as:
- seeking conflict;
- difficulty in controlling pain ('total pain');
- attention-seeking behaviour;
- complaining about the lack of information.

Fear is best treated without medicine if the necessary examination or treatment does not endanger (and is bearable for) the patient. In such cases the doctor is limited to empathetic reassurance. Behaviour therapy can be used to reinforce behaviour patterns, such as improving the patient's defence mechanisms through slow, deep breathing and relaxation techniques, particularly when faced with fear caused by the anticipation of an examination or treatment.

Treating anxiety

Debilitating physical problems must be treated and any medication that triggers these conditions should be stopped. The healthcare professional must be reassuring and encourage the patient to express their thoughts and feelings about their situation while remaining supportive and providing them with information that they may find useful. Suggested options include relaxation techniques and possibly prescribing anti-anxiety medication (see Annex, p. 222).

The loss of self-control is an extremely important factor in triggering anxiety in seriously ill patients. The treatment is therefore mainly based on restoring (insofar as it is possible) and maintaining autonomy. For this reason it is important to be careful when prescribing anxiolytics. Most of these belong to the benzodiazepine family (for example Xanax®) which have a sedative effect, and if the prescribed dose is too high can lead to further loss of control, thereby increasing rather than calming the anxiety. This can cause a vicious cycle for the patient.

Fear of death is often accompanied by numerous physical complications resulting in the loss of independence. Fear of dying is a normal part of being human: the ultimate existential question, the fear of no longer existing. Dying people can be afraid of isolation and being cut off by death. Anxiety in claustrophobic patients may even reach extreme proportions at the thought of being confined in the limited space of a coffin. This negative state of mind is often very difficult and confrontational for the family and healthcare professionals, but this is not a reason to avoid these problems by using heavy sedation. Patients must not be sedated to spare the bystanders. In many instances, another possibility is to call on spiritual assistance in the guise of a religious leader. Palliative sedation can only be considered, following consultation, when the patient gives verbal or displays non-verbal signs of unsustainable fear.

Anxiety-motivated requests for euthanasia

Requests for euthanasia are not all made by patients whose medical condition is without hope and whose suffering is unbearable. Patients often request euthanasia through fear of future suffering or loss of self-control. Giving themselves the option of euthanasia with the knowledge that they can pull the 'emergency brake' at any time is often enough to reassure patients sufficiently for them to move on; yet another reason to have a euthanasia law. In these circumstances, debating the option of euthanasia can reduce anxiety and even prolong life.

Anorexia-cachexia syndrome: the gaunt patient

Everyone knows the stereotype of an advanced cancer patient with no appetite who is reduced to skin and bone. This was previously, without much consideration, attributed to the destructive nature of the disease: the anorexia led to inadequate absorption of nutrients and calories and at the same time the fast-growing tumour took its energy needs from the patient's fat reserves, with extreme weight loss as a result.

Since then, a clearer understanding of the so-called anorexia-cachexia syndrome has been developed. The word anorexia comes from the Greek 'an' ('without') and 'orexis' ('appetite'), while the term 'cachexia' originates from 'kakos' ('bad') and 'hexis' ('condition').

A number of observations were indeed contrary to the reasoning 'not eating equals loss of weight'. On the one hand were cancer patients who, despite having healthy appetites, still lost weight, while on the other, many incurable breast-cancer patients, for example, never appear emaciated, unlike most lung-cancer patients.

Primary anorexia-cachexia syndrome is a specific entity in itself and is caused by metabolic disorders. There is an abnormal metabolism of sugars, proteins and fats leading to anorexia, emaciation (cachexia), weakness and weight loss.

This syndrome can be aggravated by all kinds of triggers. The main factors that lead to *secondary* anorexia-cachexia are listed in Table 5 below. As mentioned earlier, these secondary factors were previously considered to be the only cause of anorexia and emaciation. It is important to recognise them because they can be better treated than the actual primary anorexia-cachexia syndrome.

The feeling of weakness or fatigue in primary anorexia-cachexia should not be confused with other disorders that can cause general or local asthenia.

Local weakness is caused by peripheral nerve injuries or by a brain tumour resulting in a one-sided loss of strength (hemiparesis) or general weakening.

The causes of general weakness or fatigue (see Table 6 below) are often curable. The question, as always, is to what extent it is useful to the patient to improve them.

Primary anorexia-cachexia syndrome

Primary anorexia-cachexia syndrome has nothing to do with triggering factors referred to above or with conditions that lead to weakness or fatigue. However, it occurs frequently in advanced cancer patients and is characterised by a lack of appetite (anorexia), weight loss (cachexia) and emaciation, which in turn results in weakness (asthenia).

TABLE 5   FACTORS THAT TRIGGER ANOREXIA-CACHEXIA SYNDROME

- Eating less
    - difficulty in swallowing, caused among other things by radiotherapy
    - serious constipation
    - nausea and vomiting
    - serious pain
    - confusion
    - dry, inflamed mouth
    - taste buds affected by chemotherapy
- Reduced intake of food by the intestines due to chronic diarrhoea
- Loss of proteins
    - frequent ascites and pleural punctures
    - kidney disorder with protein loss (nephrotic syndrome)
- Muscle loss due to immobility
- Chronic infections, heart failure, lung and kidney failure, liver cirrhosis
- Psychosocial and spiritual stress

TABLE 6 GENERAL WEAKNESS

Causes	Possible treatment
Anaemia	blood transfusion
Hypercalcaemia	bisphosphonates
Hypokalemia	k-supplement
Myopathy	corticoids
Depression	counselling, anti-depressants
Chemotherapy	evaluate, maybe stop
Radiotherapy	evaluate, maybe stop
Corticoids	reduce
Diuretics	reduce
Sleeplessness	pain therapy, sleeping pills
Exhaustion	pain and symptom control
Infection	antibiotics, antipyretics
Dehydration	rehydration
Malnutrition	diet

It manifests in the abnormal metabolism of sugars, fats and proteins leading to glucose intolerance, too many fats and too little protein in the blood.

It is the leading cause of death in most cancer patients.

What is seen?

Anorexia

Anorexia leads to reduced food intake. In recent years we have come to understand that there are factors circulating in the bloodstream of cancer patients which have a significant influence on anorexia and cachexia. These factors not only cause anorexia, but are also responsible for the abnormal metabolism that has already taken hold before the syndrome manifests itself clinically.

Hunger and satiety are affected in various different ways. One important factor is the vagus nerve that sends all food-related signals – mechanical, chemical and hormonal (including cytokines, see p. 60) – from the stomach and intestinal system to the central nervous system. Another influential role is played by the melanocortin system of the epiphysis that controls the day–night rhythm. Cannabinoid receptors have also been found in the hypothalamus (the relay system for incoming signals within the central nervous system). It is thought that these are the reason why cannabis stimulates the appetite.

Abnormal metabolism

- Sugars. Increased glucose consumption and the synthesis of glucose from amino acids, the building blocks of all proteins.
- Proteins. Muscle proteins are mobilised and processed into glucose, creating a shortage of proteins resulting in: emaciation, muscle weakening, oedemas, anaemia, failure of the immune system due to the inadequate production of antibodies and bad wound healing. This is in contrast to prolonged fasting (such as was experienced by prisoners in the Nazi camps) in which fats are used up before the proteins are broken down.

- Fats. In cancer patients, the fat is broken down and normal fat distribution is disturbed, with the result that they have a build-up of fat in their blood and suffer from high cholesterol and increased triglycerides.

Weight loss

All of this ultimately leads to weight loss by muscle breakdown and reduced fat reserves.

What causes this syndrome?

Cachexia is not only caused by anorexia. Abnormal metabolisms have been seen in cancer patients who have not yet shown any signs of anorexia. Moreover, it is not always possible to reverse this syndrome through artificial feeding.

Neither can it be blamed on the higher energy needs of the growing tumour. Many human tumours have a metabolic rate that is comparable to or even lower than normal tissue.

Moreover, cachexia is dependent on the type of cancer. It occurs mainly in lung and pancreatic tumours, and much less frequently in breast cancer.

It has been suggested that certain substances that interfere with the patient's metabolism circulate in the body. Several factors were identified as potential causes of anorexia and cachexia. The most researched of these are the cytokines (see p. 60). The main cytokines responsible for cachexia are the tumour necrosis factor (aptly called 'cachectin'), Interleukin-1 (IL-1), interferon γ and to a lesser extent, IL-6.

The syndrome is caused by a complex interaction between the tumour and its 'host'. The question remains whether these substances are produced primarily by the body or by the tumour.

The tumour necrosis factor (TNF) was first discovered in rabbits infected with the trypanosoma cruzi parasite responsible for Chagas disease in South America. The rabbits developed anorexia, protein deterioration, weight loss, anaemia and inflammation. When injected into test animals it also caused bloody tissue breakdown (necrosis) of experimental tumours: hence the name 'tumour necrosis factor'. When administered to cancer patients, TNF leads to anorexia and cachexia. Cachectin is produced by certain white blood cells, such as macrophages and lymphocytes in cancer patients.

Interleukin-1 and interferon γ cause fever, inflammation, anorexia and weight loss.

Certain substances that can cause anorexia and cachexia were isolated from the tumours themselves. Proteolysis-inducing factor (PIF) is a protein that promotes the breakdown of proteins and thus damages muscle proteins.

The study of anorexia-cachexia syndrome remains complex because these substances are very difficult to detect. Cytokines act locally and are only present in the bloodstream for a limited time.

What can be done about it?

The syndrome occurs in incurable patients. The main objective is therefore to *maximise comfort* by removing:

- Trigger factors leading to the so-called secondary anorexia-cachexia, such as chronic nausea, vomiting, swallowing problems, depression and pain, which sustain the anorexia. Chronic nausea (68 per cent) is very important and has multiple causes: bowel obstruction, chemotherapy, intracranial pressure caused by brain metastases, malfunctioning of the autonomous nervous system, morphine, metabolic abnormalities such as hypercalcaemia, peptic ulcers and radiotherapy. Taking the time to explain to the patient, in language that they understand, the possible cause of their nausea is already a step in the right direction. It can help motivate them to complete chemotherapy. Food and drink is very important for most people in fuelling their zest for life.
- Asthenia is a regrettable consequence of this syndrome for which little can be done to help.
- Changed body image: clothes are now too big; eyes appear sunken in their sockets. More attention needs to be paid to these elements because they can be very depressing.

What about malnutrition and abnormal metabolism in these patients? Can their nutritional state be improved? What medication is available?

Abnormal metabolism is caused by circulating cytokines, against which there is currently very little that can be done.

Improved nutrition?

Artificial feeding through a tube or a vein has no impact on the effects and toxicity of chemo- and radiotherapy, nor on life expectancy. It is therefore important to consider whether it is worth pursuing this option. Once started, it is very difficult to stop for psychological reasons.

There are, however, situations where temporary tube-feeding can be useful for incurable patients. It can help wounds heal better as well as prevent infections and other complications after surgery. Reduced food intake as a result of temporary swallowing problems following radiotherapy for head and neck tumours can be counteracted in this way.

Artificial feeding is by no means superior to oral feeding. Being referred to hospital for intravenous hyperalimentation is therefore out of the question. It has no impact on the patient's general comfort levels such as physical symptoms or general fitness.

Should patients be encouraged to eat more? Following a particular diet only has an effect for three weeks. It is more important to convince the family that 'forcing' the patient to eat more has little influence on their comfort levels and can even have a negative impact, and frequently leads to frustrations on both sides. The family is unhappy because the patient pushes aside a 'delicious' stew, whereas the patient feels nauseated and feels depressed because they feel they are letting their family and friends down. Nevertheless it is still very difficult to move past the maxim 'food is healthy'. This is not only to do with the impending end and the idea of separation. Food and drink are among the few things that friends can still do for incurable patients. The healthcare professional should therefore suggest acceptable alternatives: prepare frequent but small snacks to give the patient when they feel like it: ice cream, beer, cookies, champagne. Traditional health concerns such as 'Can they have a glass of wine?' do not apply in these instances. Even if the patient is on morphine, the only danger is that they will sleep longer or better.

Medication?

Medicines which have proved to be effective are metoclopramide (Primperan®), corticoids and progestins. Products with a potential value are thalidomide, anabolic steroids, cannabinoids, melatonin, growth hormone, omega-3 fatty acids and NSAIDs. Useless resources are cyproheptadine and hydrazine sulphate (see Annex, p. 222).

Conclusion

It is a complex syndrome, the cause of which is still not well known. Consequently, there are few therapeutic options available. Artificial feeding makes little sense, except to combat acute problems.

Medicines can be tested using metoclopramide, corticoids (short-term effect) or progestins (longer-term effect). It is of the utmost importance to support the patient and their family, as is improving their general comfort, whereas any weight gain is not. Scales ought to be banned.

Dyspnea

Dyspnea, or tightness of chest and shortness of breath, is a subjective sensation. It is the feeling of having difficulty breathing: the inability to breathe 'deeply', which may result in choking, followed by acute anxiety attacks. This subjective sensation is in stark contrast to the more objective oxygen deprivation (hypoxia) with cyanosis (blue discoloration) of the skin, lips, earlobes and the nail bed due to the increased amount of reduced haemoglobin (low oxygen saturation).

It should not be confused with accelerated breathing caused by fever (tachypnea), 'heavy' breathing caused by diabetic ketoacidosis (Kussmaul breathing) and the shallow breathing (hyperventilation) provoked by various psychological factors such as anxiety. It is striking that 80 per cent of all lung cancer patients in the course of their illness exhibit some form of dyspnea.

Table 7 below gives some problems that can provoke dyspnea and possible interventions to counter them.

In such cases, it is, as always, important to consult with the patient in deciding whether corrective measures will deliver more advantages than disadvantages. Does it make sense to treat pneumonia in a bed-ridden, emaciated, 40 kg patient who no can longer eat or drink with antibiotics?

Many of these problems, in advanced stages, can give rise to a real lack of oxygen.

Oxygen: a burdensome placebo for dyspnea

In cases of purely subjective difficulty in breathing (without real oxygen deprivation – recognisable by cyanosis), oxygen is too often administered as 'therapy'. This is very dangerous because the placebo effect of oxygen is huge. It is known that, once administered, the patient with difficulty breathing will struggle to do so without oxygen, especially in periods of serious lung problems. In addition, it is a not insignificant burden for the home-care team to require that a supply of oxygen bottles be on hand.

It is therefore better to reserve oxygen treatment for emergencies such as hypoxia. Morphine preparations or substances such as alprazolam (Xanax®) can often be effective in treating dyspnea (see Annex, p. 223).

TABLE 7   CAUSES OF DYSPNEA

Pleural effusion	puncture
Bronchial obstruction	laser, stent, radiotherapy
Infection	antibiotics
Lymphangitis	corticoids, radiotherapy
Reduced lung volume (for example lobectomy)	corticoids
Emboly	anti-coagulants
Radiation fibrosis	corticoids, opiates
Vena cava superior syndrome	corticoids, radiotherapy
Abdominal distension (e.g. ascites)	depending on the cause (for example puncture)
Anaemia (e.g. bone marrow invasion)	for example transfusion
Cardiac (for example pulmonary oedema)	depending on the cause (for example digitalis, opiates, diuretics)

Constipation

Difficult bowel movements are very common, especially in inactive, bedridden patients with reduced appetites who only eat small quantities of fresh fruit or vegetables and who drink too little. Most healthy people have on average five to seven bowel movements a week. The same frequency cannot be expected from seriously ill patients on medication with constipating side-effects. Nevertheless it is important to look out for constipation and try to avoid solid, immobile faeces (faecal impaction) and all its consequences.

Another pitfall is the masking of advanced constipation by so-called 'overflow-diarrhoea'. Bacteria from the intestinal flora 'soften' the upper part of the solid stool into a slimy liquid that then seeps down the side of the stool and out of the anus. These secretions can be incorrectly viewed as diarrhoea.

The immediate response to reduced bowel movements or constipation is to blame it on morphine preparations (it is almost professional misconduct to treat a patient with morphine without adding a laxative) but other frequently prescribed medications also make bowel movements difficult, especially when administered together: some NSAIDs, tricyclic antidepressants, antihistamines, antiemetics, neuroleptics and certain chemotherapy drugs such as vincristine (Oncovin®). Metabolic abnormalities such as hypercalcaemia, hypokalemia and deregulated diabetes can cause constipation.

Constipation can also be caused by patient-related factors such as inactivity and being bedridden, pressure ulcers, fever, decreased food and fluid intake, ascites, digestive and brain tumours, spinal-cord injuries, haemorrhoids and anal fissures. These factors are, however, usually harder to deal with.

Constipation can be quickly diagnosed by palpation of the abdomen and a 'rectal examination'. For the treatment and prevention of constipation refer to the Annex (see p. 224).

Delirium

Delirium or acute confusion is caused by an organic brain dysfunction and is characterised by a disruption to cognitive functions (perception, attention, memory, orientation, language skills) and psychomotor functions associated with agitation, drowsiness, hallucinations and delusions.

Most cancer patients, but also other patients, experience this in their last week, although some also experience a number of reversible episodes of delirium before this.

It is a very important problem, given that the diagnosis is often missed, especially during the initial stages. Early symptoms such as anxiety, panic, insomnia and behaviour disorders are incorrectly treated with anxiolytics or antidepressants which can exacerbate the delirium.

It can manifest as acute or sub-acute, possibly with a fluctuating course.

Delirium can be either hyperactive (confusion and agitation with hallucinations and delusions) or hypoactive (confusion and somnolence) or a combination of the two. This makes the diagnosis difficult.

Hypoactive delirium is often mistaken for depression or dementia. In advanced cancer patients there are far more instances of delirium (up to 80 per cent) than depression (10 per cent). Dementia usually sets in earlier or concerns patients over eighty.

Psychomotor activity may or may not increase: perspiration, palpitations, pupil dilation, restlessness and dry mouth.

Delirium can be caused by several factors.

Where possible, and if it still makes sense, the underlying cause should be corrected.

Things to consider include:

- Medicines

  Morphine toxicity (pupil constriction); consider an opioid rotation. Other medication: such as benzodiazepines, antiemetics, anticholinergic agents (pupil dilation), anticonvulsants, antidepressants, corticoids (muscle aches and joint pain), NSAIDs, methylphenidate and alcohol. Abstinence can also cause this: benzodiazepines, opioids, nicotine and alcohol.

- Dehydration: If no intravenous rehydration with a physiological solution is possible, consider using a hypodermoclysis (a subcutaneous infusion of 60–100 ml per hour or boluses of 500 ml per hour to be repeated three or four times).

- Hypercalcaemia: treat with bisphosphonates (Zometa®).
- Hypoxia (dyspnea; tachypnea): treat if possible (for example blood transfusion) and supply oxygen.
- Intracranial problems: brain tumour or metastases, brain haemorrhage, carcinomatous meningitis, etc.
- Generalised infections (low blood pressure; tachycardia): consider starting antibiotics.
- Kidney or liver disease ('flapping tremor') or other metabolic disorders such as dehydration, blood-sugar abnormalities (hypo: clamminess, cold; hyper: dry, hot).
- Chemotherapy or radiotherapy.

Delirium can also be provoked or aggravated by anxiety, depression, pain, physical discomfort such as urinary retention or constipation, sleep deprivation or a changed environment such as hospitalisation or existing dementia.

In addition to a possible cure for the underlying causes of delirium, the symptoms can also be treated with medication (see Annex, p. 225).

Another element to bear in mind is the general reception, and the importance of a quiet, well-lit area, of not being strapped to the bed or bedrails, of limiting the number of strange faces and the presence of familiar faces and close friends, a regular daily routine and a calm demeanour and clear explanations when possible. Allowing (moderate) use of tobacco and alcohol cannot be underestimated.

One of the characteristics of a delirium is the loss of inhibition, both verbal and non-verbal. This needs to be well monitored as it can be very stressful for onlookers. Examples of non-verbal disinhibition are making grimaces or moaning without physical discomfort. If wrongly interpreted, more morphine or benzodiazepines may be prescribed, thereby exacerbating the delirium. Verbal examples of disinhibition are expressions such as 'I want to go home now.' Again it is important to give a clear explanation to the family to avoid feelings of guilt.

Terminal agitation: the delirium of the last days of life

This delirium is characterised by agitated, restless behaviour, shouting out, impeded consciousness, twitching and multifocal myoclonus and sometimes even convulsions.

In such instances, the other reasons for agitation should also be excluded:

- fear of death/agony;
- pain;
- urinary retention, faecal impaction;
- abstinence from medicines, alcohol or nicotine.

Terminal agitation is mainly treated using medicamentous therapy (see Annex, p. 225).

Depression

Being diagnosed with a potentially life-threatening condition such as cancer and all its consequences can provoke a violent emotional upheaval. Fortunately this feeling of abject distress is transient for most patients and, with the necessary support, can be overcome by both the patient and family. Nevertheless, about a third of cancer patients suffer from mild 'depression' and 10 per cent experience serious depression.

In practice, it is very difficult to diagnose seriously ill patients with depression with any certainty, not least because it makes sense for them to be sad and grieving. The DSM-V classification is therefore used in diagnosing depression. In order to be able to speak of a major depressive episode, five or more of the following symptoms must be present almost every day for at least two weeks:

- a depressed mood for the greater part of the day;
- a decreased interest or pleasure in most daily activities;
- a more than 5 per cent weight loss or gain in a month, or reduced (or increased) appetite;
- insomnia or lethargy;
- psychomotor agitation or retardation;
- fatigue or loss of energy;

- a sense of worthlessness or guilt;
- reduced ability to think or concentrate, indecisiveness;
- recurrent thoughts about death or suicidal tendencies.

At least one of the first two symptoms must be present (depressed mood and decreased interest or pleasure).

The main problem, however, is that the symptoms mentioned above, such as fatigue, anorexia and insomnia can also be caused by the disease as a result of anaemia, hypercalcaemia or poorly controlled pain, among other things.

In addition, medication given to critically ill patients such as corticoids, anticonvulsants, pain-relievers and interferon can give the impression of depression and even trigger the same symptoms as a major depressive episode.

It remains a very difficult diagnosis. The following pointers may be helpful in identifying and dealing with a major depressive episode in a seriously ill patient:

- Has the patient exhibited signs of depressive periods prior to their illness, or is there a history of depression or suicide in the family?
- Exclude delirium (see p. 106).
- Ask the patient if they have ever considered suicide.
- Spend time with the patient during the follow-up: short but frequent interventions are better than long irregular visits.
- Create the right environment for recovery: the patient should be comfortable and possibly accompanied by well-wishers.
- Gain trust by being empathic without creating unrealistic expectations.

The role of antidepressants in patients with life-threatening conditions

Although the optimal use of antidepressants in cancer patients is not clear, various observations suggest that they can be useful in certain patients (see Annex, p. 218).

Requests for euthanasia and depression

Some people still argue that seriously ill patients should not be allowed to ask for euthanasia because they are 'depressive' due to their illness and can no longer be considered to be in a fit state to make this kind of decision. We have already demonstrated that the majority of cancer patients do not experience major depression. Most patients feel immense sadness when they realise that they are seriously, even terminally ill, thinking about what is ahead of them: saying goodbye to life and family, a lesser quality of life, separation, losing everything and dying. This sadness is not to be confused with major depression. Non-depressed patients, for example, say that they have had a fantastic life, but are now sad at what is to happen.

A request for euthanasia necessarily requires insight into the patient's psychopathology; yet another argument in favour of an interdisciplinary solution. When in doubt ask the advice of a psychologist.

Nausea and vomiting

Vomiting, gagging and nausea are very unpleasant and can even be unbearable. They are common in seriously ill people. The following schematic representation is useful in the selection of certain anti-vomiting agents. Unfortunately, the causes are often multiple and not always easy to figure out. Luckily some anti-emetics target many causes, which may explain their success in various circumstances.

Aetiology

Nausea is an extremely unpleasant sensation in the upper part of the digestive system and is often accompanied by an urge to vomit. This gagging can be described as rhythmic spasmodic movements of the diaphragm and abdominal muscles in the presence of nausea. Gagging often precedes vomiting and sometimes the two alternate.

Nausea is caused by stimulation of the autonomic nervous system, linking it to other autonomous symptoms such as pallor (going white), cold sweats, salivation, palpitations and even diarrhoea.

Vomiting follows the stimulation of the 'emetic centre', a specialised region of the central nervous system located on the medulla oblongata (spinal cord just below the skull).

The emetic centre can be stimulated in four ways: from the cerebral cortex, the vestibular system (via the vestibular nuclei in the brainstem), from the 'chemoreceptor trigger zone' and finally by peripheral nerves (see Figure 3).

Stimuli from the central nervous system can as easily be of psychological as organic origin. Psychogenic vomiting by patients who enter the chemotherapy department is well known. Anxiety and pain can also cause a patient to throw up. Finally, any cause of increased pressure in the skull can cause massive vomiting: increased blood pressure, coughing, brain metastases etc.

FIGURE 3   STIMULATION OF THE EMETIC CENTRE

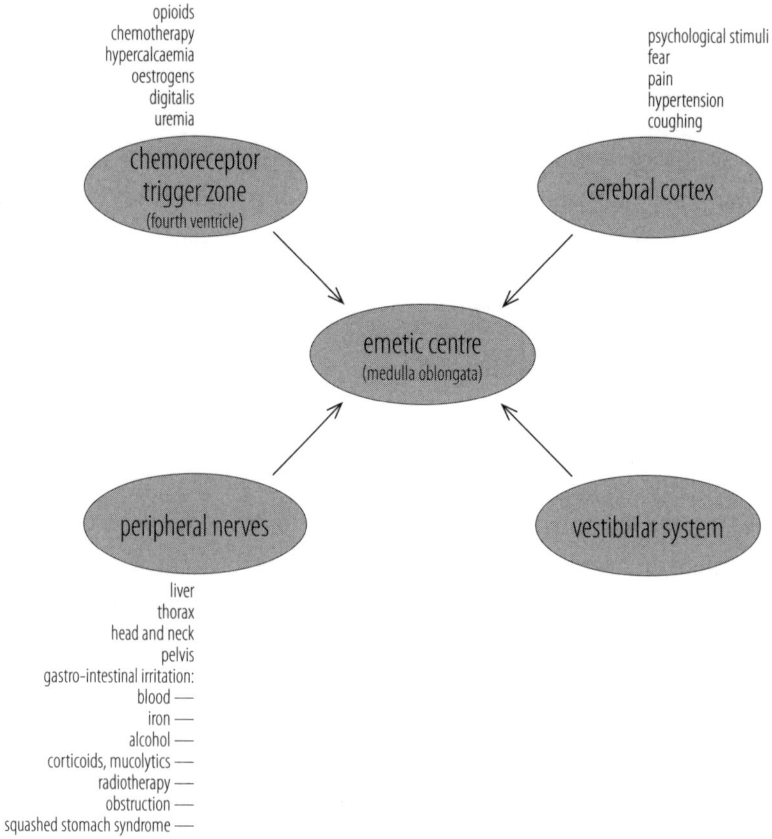

The 'chemoreceptor trigger zone' (CTZ) consists of highly specialised cells and is located in the so-called area postrema at the bottom of the fourth ventricle in the brain stem. These cells are highly sensitive to concentrations of certain substances in the blood, such as opioids, chemotherapeutic agents, increased concentration of oestrogens in pregnancy, hypercalcaemia from bone metastases, hyponatremia, uraemia from renal failure and digitalis preparations administered for heart failure. The area postrema also generates stimuli from the vestibular system which can explain the nausea and possibly vomiting from car- and sea-sickness, and the vagus nerve also sends stimuli from the gastrointestinal tract. Motion sickness is of course less relevant for seriously ill patients.

Peripheral nerves can be stimulated by irritation of the gastrointestinal system, for example from a stomach ulcer or gastritis, blood stasis in the stomach, other irritating influences on the gastric mucosa such as corticoids, NSAIDs, mucolytics, alcohol, iron preparations, local radiotherapy, constipation caused by hard stools and bowel obstruction or the squashed stomach syndrome where the stomach is flattened by abdominal distention caused by ascites fluid.

Peripheral nerves in other regions can also lead to vomiting: stimulation of the lung pleura, the pelvis, the head and neck area and the liver. Vomiting is often the first sign of liver metastasis. The liver tissue feels no pain but the enlarged liver (from tumour oedema) exerts painful pressure on the rigid liver capsule, resulting in a dull pain right below the ribs, causing vomiting. In such cases, trial therapy with corticoids can often provoke a spectacular result in a very short time, both for the pain and the vomiting.

The diagram is helpful in choosing an anti-vomiting drug. Receptors for the same drug can often be found at various levels. This explains why the same product works for different causes of vomiting (see Annex, p. 226).

In addition to the medication there are general measures that should be taken as they are often effective as a preventive measure. Provide the patient with:

- a quiet area, away from the smell and the sight of food;
- many small snacks, rather than one elaborate meal;

- treatment for reversible causes such as coughing, constipation, hypercalcaemia etc.;
- withdrawal of any drugs that irritate the stomach, like corticoids, antibiotics or NSAIDs etc.

Less common symptoms

Some annoying problems are less common but the patient experiencing these symptoms doesn't and shouldn't therefore expect less help. A selection of these is listed here.

Ascites

Ascites is an abnormal build-up of fluid in the abdominal cavity. It is often caused by obstruction of the main veins in the abdomen: the lower hollow vein and the hepatic vein (vena hepatica). This in turn obstructs the reflux of blood to the heart and fluid seeps into the abdomen. The most common cause is liver cirrhosis, but also liver metastasis. Diffuse metastases in the abdominal cavity itself can also cause ascites.

A distended belly can be very difficult and lead to:
- anorexia, acid indigestion, nausea and vomiting;
- shortness of breath;
- ankle oedema;
- fatigue.

When it becomes too much for the patient, it is possible to relieve the pressure by draining the fluid. This is a very simple procedure that can be done at home, or in a palliative day-care unit.

Bladder spasms and bladder irritation

Bladder irritation can be caused by:
- a (clogged) catheter;
- infection (cystitis);
- a bladder tumour or a tumour in the pelvic region;
- irradiation of the bladder region;

- chemotherapy of the bladder;
- urinary retention: blocked by a kidney stone.

Treatment depends on the cause: antibiotics for infection, a catheter for urinary retention and possibly painkillers as well as drugs to relieve the bladder spasms (see Annex, p. 227).

Diarrhoea

In this section we are not talking about the acute diarrhoea caused by a digestive infection which is limited in time. Diarrhoea only becomes a real problem when it is persistent. We speak of chronic diarrhoea when it lasts longer than three weeks with a real danger of dehydration, especially in older patients.

Chronic diarrhoea in cancer patients is caused by:

- medication: laxatives, certain NSAIDs, diuretics, certain anti-depressants and antibiotics;
- a paradoxical reaction to a partial obstruction of the intestine by a tumour;
- poor digestion due to aberrant production of hormones by specific tumours in the stomach or intestine system, pancreatic tumours or carcinoid tumours;
- therapeutic ablation of the coeliacus nerve plexus (to relieve pain);
- feeding tubes;
- after 'active' treatment:
  - radiotherapy;
  - chemotherapy, especially with cisplatin, irinotecan or 5-fluorouracil;
  - surgery after removing a large piece of intestine (short bowel syndrome) or an ileostomy;
  - immune response after allogeneic bone-marrow transplantation (graft versus host disease).

Insofar as it is possible, the aim should always be to eliminate the cause. Treating and preventing dehydration is also very important: the patient should drink a lot – soft drinks are good – but avoid bowel-stimulating ingredients such as alcohol, coffee, carbonated beverages (shake any carbonated drinks to reduce the gas), onions and cabbage. Anti-diarrhoea pills may offer temporary relief. An Imodium® tablet can be administered after each loose bowel movement up to eight times a day (see Annex, p. 227).

Bowel obstruction

Complete bowel obstruction can occur at one time or another in patients with bowel cancer. It is also possible with other conditions such as ovarian cancer with metastasis.

A surgeon will first treat a bowel obstruction caused by an acute condition such as acute appendicitis using the drip and suck technique: a drip to prevent dehydration and a tube in the stomach to remove (suck) the intestinal moisture while waiting for surgical intervention. Again, it is questionable whether this treatment makes sense for a terminal patient who can no longer undergo surgery. In addition, the stomach tube, once installed, has to stay there, which is very cumbersome and doesn't improve oral communication.

In such cases, after thorough consideration, it may be better to adopt a more conservative attitude and fight the symptoms with drugs (see Annex, p. 224).

Hiccups

Hiccups are an automatic reflex of the muscles in the diaphragm and thorax. Persistent hiccups become unbearable.

Hiccups are caused by irritations to the brainstem, the central part of the brain or various nerves (including the phrenic nerve in the diaphragm, the vagus nerve in the gastrointestinal tract, the recurrent nerve and even the intercostal nerves). The hiccup reflex can occur at all of these levels.

Hiccups are mainly caused by stomach distention with delayed emptying. Other causes are:
- underlying abdominal tumours, an enlarged liver, ascites;
- problems in the oesophagus, such as reflux or inflammation;
- infection of the lung base;

- tumours or inflammation of the brain or brain stem;
- metabolic disorders: hypernatremia, hypercalcaemia , uremia;
- certain medications: benzodiazepines, barbiturates, etoposide;
- alcohol abuse.

For treatment, see Annex, p. 228.

Coughing

Coughing is a complex reflex of the airways to remove foreign materials and excess mucus. Any irritation in the airways makes a person cough – not only infections but also chronic bronchitis and asthma, smoke, dry air, heart failure, psychological stimuli and choking. Complications from lung cancer or lung metastases cause coughing, as does irradiation of the lungs.

Underlying causes must be corrected: antibiotics for severe infections, bronchodilation for asthma, a ban on smoking, diuretics for heart failure. If possible, the mechanical irritation of the respiratory tract should be treated with aspiration, irradiation, chemotherapy, trial therapy with corticoids, laser treatment or inserting a stent.

Placing a humidifier in the room can work wonders. It helps loosen the dried mucus and makes it easier to cough up.

Most commercial cough syrups contain *undersized* doses of anti-cough medicine, a mucolytic agent, a sympathomimetic drug and an antihistamine. The main component of these syrups is usually the soothing effect of the syrup itself on the lining of the throat. Cough sweets work in the same way. Certain medicines can be administered for a persistent cough (see Annex, p. 229)

Itching

Itching is caused by many factors and can be unbearable. It is common in malignant blood diseases such as Hodgkin's disease, non-Hodgkin's lymphomas, multiple myeloma and leukaemia. Certain tumours also exhibit itching as a paraneoplastic phenomenon. Obstruction of the bile duct or cholestasis can also cause itching. This is because the bile salts are no longer secreted in the intestine but in the blood stream. Finally, certain drugs cause itching:

- via cholestasis: contraceptives, ketoconazole (Nizoral®);
- via the release of histamine: opioids.

Certain factors can exacerbate the itching:

- dry skin;
- damage to the skin: raw cotton clothing;
- sweating;
- wet skin;
- nervousness and fear.

Good skincare is therefore primary. Some medication can also help. And finally, a regular bath with 'starch' (amylum) can offer enormous relief. (see Annex, p. 229).

Oedemas

Lymphoedema is a swelling of the tissues, for example in the limbs, due to a build-up of protein-rich fluid as a result of clogged drainage through the lymph vessels. This obstruction can be caused by the growth of a tumour or metastases in the lymph vessels or lymph nodes. The lymph drainage may also have been impeded by a surgical procedure or after radiotherapy, such as after a mastectomy and supplementary irradiation.

Once the lymphoedema has formed it can never be completely healed. As the protein fibres settle, the oedema becomes hard as a result of fibrosis. It is best treated as early as possible for maximum improvement. Moisture-wicking materials (which have general fluid-retention properties) appear to have a limited impact except if the oedema is exacerbated after treatment with corticoids or NSAIDs. These drugs give rise to a generalised fluid retention. Corticoids can, however, be used to reduce the localised obstruction of the lymph nodes by tumour-infiltration.

Lymphoedema are also very susceptible to infection and can lead to life-threatening cellulitis. Small cuts in the oedematous region must therefore be avoided if possible and even treated anticipatively with antibiotics.

Pleural effusion

A pleural puncture can offer a barely mobile patient enormous relief particularly when they are extremely short of breath due to a pronounced infiltration of fluid between the two lung pleura. This is an easy procedure and can be performed at home or at a nearby palliative day-care unit (see Annex, p. 229).

Attention to detail: the secret of empathy

The nurse plops the tray down on the bedside table and disappears without checking whether the patient is in a position to eat without help. The family comes to visit with a homemade pungent pig's heart broth to strengthen the patient. The doctor enters the room with a face like the grim reaper and barely says a word. The weak, bedridden AIDS patient whispers the word 'euthanasia' but the healthcare professional pretends not to hear. The overprotective, highly perfumed volunteer invades the patient's personal space to such a degree that they are repulsed by her well-meaning attention and penetrating odour. The palliative-care unit is designed in such a way that the patient cannot see out of the window.

Seriously ill people are hypersensitive to such details because they have already made so many concessions and are in an extremely weak position. The slightest improvement in their daily routine that gives them a sense of being alive is hugely appreciated.

In the introduction to 'Pain and symptom control' (see p. 81) I mention that in addition to the 'purely' medical, nursing and psychosocial arsenal there are also many small remedies that have an enormous impact on the quality of life of seriously ill patients.

These include things such as avoiding annoying routines like taking the patient's blood pressure at 7 a.m. every morning, to using high-impact little 'tricks' such as placing pieces of sheepskin under the heels to prevent bedsores.

The possibilities are endless and depend only on the degree of experience and ingenuity of the interdisciplinary team: healthcare professionals, volunteers, family and other loved ones.

The importance of empathy cannot be underestimated. Empathy is not the same as pity. Pity creates distance and emphasises the difference in fate. Empathy means seeing things through the patient's eyes, hearing with their ears and thinking with their brain.

As an example, here are some suggestions about oral hygiene which patients tend to really appreciate. The mouth is important because basic needs such as food and drink become very important in precarious situations. Key areas for attention tend to be related to sensory perception and basic needs, such as hearing, smell, sight, touch and being manipulated, urination and bowel movements, breathing, sleeping and lying comfortably and the skin.

Poor oral hygiene not only means less consumption of food and water but also difficulties in verbal communication. Regular attention to the mouth can avoid much misery.

Keep the lips smooth and avoid (the threat of) dehydration: petroleum jelly, cocoa butter.

The oral cavity itself can become dehydrated. This is often caused by certain drugs (morphine, benzodiazepines, antidepressants, antidiarreïca, and diuretics) or after irradiation.

It is important to encourage the patient to eat and drink a lot and to keep the air moist with a humidifier. In the final phase it becomes difficult to drink. The patient may feel thirsty but that is mainly due to the dryness in the mouth itself. This can be alleviated by dabbing the local area with a wet washcloth or giving the patient ice cubes (crushed or not) to suck on – if so desired these can be made from fresh oranges. This also helps to ease the pain. Other options for keeping the mouth clean and soft (for example in the event of inflammation) are: yogurt on the tongue, chamomile tea or Kamillosan (1–2 teaspoons in a glass of water), Isobetadine mouth rinse (diluted 1:1 in water). Painful ulcerations after radiotherapy or cancer sores respond well to prepared solutions (see Annex, p. 208).

Pineapple chunks can be used to clean the mouth, and tongue seizures or scabs can be removed with cola or oxygen water. One can also give the patient a vitamin C tablet (Redoxon®) to melt on the tongue.

Emergencies

Even incurable patients experience emergencies, the symptoms of which if recognised in time and treated can be properly controlled. These include spinal-cord compression from vertebral metastases, brain metastases, superior vena cava syndrome, hypercalcaemia and massive haemorrhaging from the gradual eating away of an artery. Apart from the hypercalcaemia and the haemorrhaging, these emergencies can mostly be treated in the same way: high doses of corticoids possibly followed by irradiation (see Annex, p. 230).

Spinal-cord compression by spinal metastases

It is important to be alert to comments such as 'I have back pain after working in the garden', especially from patients with oncological history. They may be the first symptoms of spinal metastases with infiltration in the inter-vertebral space and damage to the nerves. If overlooked, this can result in emotional disorders, muscle weakness and even paralysis of the legs and urinary and/or rectal incontinence. It is irresponsible to let someone die paralysed when it can be prevented.

The treatment is immediately to reduce any swelling by administering corticoids.

If the prognosis reveals that the patient's condition is still reasonable, radiotherapy or surgical decompression by laminectomy can be considered. Both treatments have equal value. If, however, the paralysis gets worse during radiotherapy, it must be stopped immediately and a switch made to a laminectomy.

The neurological status before treatment is extremely important in the prognosis and chances of survival. The vast majority of patients who were still mobile before radiotherapy will fortunately stay mobile, just under half of lame patients will become mobile again, and only a few per cent of the lame ever recover (fully).

Brain metastases

Cerebral metastases occur very often. They affect up to a third of all cancer patients and are the cause of their deaths. Most of these patients exhibit neurological symptoms such as headaches, double vision, cognitive dysfunction, convulsions or motor and/or sensory loss. A CT or NMR brain scan will confirm the diagnosis.

Treatment in these cases is with corticoids to counter the cerebral oedema. The effect is visible within 24 hours, and in half of the patients the symptoms disappear spectacularly. Total brain radiotherapy can be considered, or localised irradiation on small metastases can be performed in specialised radiation treatment centres with extremely accurate radiation beams, or surgical removal.

Superior vena cava syndrome

The upper hollow vein or superior vena cava carries blood from the head, the neck, the upper part of the chest and the arms back to the heart. Lung cancer or lymphomas in this region (primarily) can cause external compression or intracaval thrombus of this vein. This, in turn, prevents the flow of blood back to the heart due to fluid build-up in the areas mentioned above. The condition can manifest in cerebral oedema with headaches and dizziness, violent dyspnea, sometimes even cyanosis, venous distension in the neck and upper thorax and facial oedema with bulging eyes and/or arms. Urgent treatment may be required for patients with oedema of the larynx to avoid choking.

Treatment consists of oxygen, radiotherapy and possibly chemotherapy in responsive tumours such as lymphoma. Inserting a stent can often provide immediate assistance. In most cases, these treatments provide relief for considerable periods. The role of corticoids in these cases is less clear, although a trial therapy is usually worth trying.

Massive haemorrhaging

Serious but not acute bleeding of the stomach and intestines, the lungs and urinary tract can often be treated with good palliative local radiotherapy.

Massive acute haemorrhages occur most often due to erosion of the carotid artery by a tumour in the head and neck area. The haemorrhages are often sudden, quick, spectacular and usually fatal. The patient quickly becomes comatose from lack of oxygen in the brain. Nevertheless, it is important to be prepared for such an eventuality for the sake of the family: discretely ensure that dark-coloured cloths are accessible, and explain tactfully what to expect and keep medicines on hand (see Annex, p. 230).

Hypercalcaemia

Hypercalcaemia is a life-threatening condition in advanced cancer. Up to one in five cancers lead to an increase of calcium in the blood.

Hypercalcaemia is a paraneoplastic syndrome caused by tumour production by the parathyroid hormone–like peptide. Like the parathyroid hormone in the parathyroid gland, this paraneoplastic substance activates the osteoclasts (cells responsible for bone resorption) with the release of calcium into the bloodstream and hypercalcaemia as a result. In addition, calcium reabsorption by the kidneys is also activated. In less common instances, the increased calcemia is the result of direct bone destruction caused by metastatic encroachments.

It occurs frequently in:

- breast cancer;
- lung cancer of squamous cell type;
- multiple myeloma;
- genito-urinary cancers;
- squamous cell carcinoma of the head and neck region.

It is rare in:

- prostate cancer;
- adenocarcinoma of the colon or stomach;
- small-cell lung cancer.

Diagnosis

These symptoms may be very unobtrusive, but manifest progressively:

- anorexia;
- vomiting and nausea;
- constipation;
- dehydration;
- polyuria (frequent urination);
- weakness and fatigue;
- confusion;
- coma.

It frequently manifests with a single isolated symptom such as constipation at the beginning, making it very difficult to make an early diagnosis.

The active component is the free ionised calcium, which accounts for almost half of the total plasma concentration. Calcium is closely bound to plasma proteins. When there are fewer plasma proteins, as with cases of pronounced cachexia, there will be relatively more free calcium available with hypercalcaemia symptoms.

Hypercalcaemia is therefore relative, and dependent on the concentration of plasma proteins. Hence it is assessed using clinical symptoms. It is possible for gradually established chronic hypercalcaemia to be fairly well tolerated.

Treatment includes rehydration (1–3 litres of physiological water per day), which helps normalise milder forms of the disease. Bisphosphonates such as Zometa® inhibit osteoclasts and thus bone resorption.

The final moments, the syringe driver's bad reputation and the problem with palliative sedation

Even when the patient is in the process of dying, it is important to remain alert to problems that can still be resolved. With the patient less alert, there is a tendency to talk loudly and frankly about their situation. This must be avoided. Patients are often still capable of following snatches of conversation.

There is the question of whether certain drugs ought to be stopped, such as those for high blood pressure. When the patient is no longer able to swallow the necessary medicines, it is possible to administer them via a subcutaneous syringe driver.

The death rattle

The dying often develop very noisy, raspy breathing. This is caused by a partial obstruction of the upper airways. When their heads are lying back on the pillow, their tongues may tilt backwards and obstruct the airways. This can be avoided by turning their heads sideways. Another possible cause is dry mucus in the upper respiratory tract that the weakened patient can no longer cough up. It slides up and down with each breath and can result in noisy vibrations. It is sometimes possible to remove this mucus with an aspiration tube although it is better to try and prevent it from forming with products that reduce mucus production (see Annex, p. 230).

Dying patients tend not to be troubled by these noises because they are often in a (sub-)comatose state. It is more of a problem for onlookers.

Why does the syringe driver have such a bad reputation?

Many people question the use of a syringe driver because they are often used for the first time during the dying phase. When the bedridden patient sinks into a coma and dies a few hours later, it is easy to link the cause of death to the pump. Below is an explanation of how the syringe driver works.

I will try and provide some clarity on this issue.

A syringe driver pumps drugs into the patient's body by means of a subcutaneous needle. This 'pain pump' can contain three types of products (see Annex, pp. 208–10):

1. drugs that have no impact on consciousness or life expectancy, even in exaggerated doses, for example corticoids;
2. products that do have an impact on consciousness or life expectancy when taken in overdose, for example morphine;
3. products whose main effect is to reduce consciousness, for example midazolam (Dormicum®).

In terms of shortening a patient's life, the only drugs of interest are those in categories 2 and 3.

There are three possible scenarios with category 2 products such as morphine:

a. The amount of product (dose) is *proportional* to the symptom. In cases of extreme dyspnea, the morphine dose must be adjusted to ensure the progressive dyspnea is bearable for the patient. If there is no life-shortening intention, it is better to under- rather than overdose with the risk that the shortness of breath is not fully cured but neither is there a risk that it will shorten the patient's life.

b. The dose is *not strictly proportional* to the symptomatology. In the previous example, the dose is not strictly monitored. It is considered better to give too much rather than too little. The condition is completely cured but there is a risk that it may shorten the patient's life.

c. A clear overdose is administered with the intention of shortening the patient's life. This can be described as 'symptom control' to the outside world, although the intention is clearly different.

Strictly speaking, the patient does not have to be consulted for options (a) and (b) – they belong officially to what is termed 'good medical practice'. If, on the other hand, the healthcare professional opts for option c without consulting the patient, it is referred to as 'life termination without request/consent'. If the patient has given their consent it is in fact euthanasia, although morphine is not normally used as a euthanaticum.

It is clear that it is possible in these situations to end a person's life without being held accountable.

The issue becomes even cloudier when the patient is sedated with products from category 3. When physical or psychological symptoms become both unbearable and untreatable it is possible to sedate the patient so that they become unconscious and are no longer aware of any suffering. This is called controlled sedation, terminal sedation or more recently palliative sedation.

Again it is possible to distinguish between the following scenarios:

a. The dose is *proportional* to the symptoms. In cases of extreme fear of death the healthcare professional will gradually increase the dose of consciousness-reducing sedatives until the patient is no longer aware of fear. If there is no life-shortening intention, it is considered better to under- rather than overdose with the risk that the fear will not totally disappear but neither is there a risk that it will shorten the patient's life.

b. The dose is *not strictly proportional* to the symptomalogy. In the previous example, the dose is not strictly monitored. It is better to over- rather than under-dose. The fear disappears completely but there is a risk that it may shorten the patient's life.

c. A clear overdose is administered with the intention of shortening the patient's life. This can be described as 'symptom control' to the outside world, although the intention is clearly different.

If the aim of palliative sedation is purely to remove the refractory symptoms and not shorten the patient's life, then option (a) is the obvious choice. Choice (b) might, but not necessarily, shorten the patient's life. These two options can be decided with or without the knowledge of the patient. Option (c) is without a doubt life-shortening without request, or euthanasia if the patient was involved in the decision.

In all these cases the interaction with any other products in the pump must be taken into account.

This reasoning obviously also applies when the drugs are not administered via a syringe driver but through a drip (a 'baxter') directly into the vein. This is usually the method used in hospital.

In daily practice, many of the situations referred to above fall under the heading 'palliative sedation'. Nevertheless it remains a nebulous 'twilight zone', allowing doctors to avoid societal control. Imagine, for example, a doctor who is not aware of all the possibilities of palliative care and incorrectly decides that a given condition is untreatable and so unilaterally decides to sedate the patient. Although this is usually done to help the patient end their life in a dignified manner, it deprives the patient or their family of the chance to say goodbye.

Inserting a syringe driver is in itself a 'neutral act' but it can cause extreme *malaise* for onlookers when the patient experiences a sudden reduction in consciousness for no apparent reason. Open and clear communication can remove doubts and prejudices about the pump.

In early 2011, there was a lot of hype around Phara De Aguirre's poignant report broadcast on Flemish television. It followed Bart Verbeeck, a young man with terminal bone cancer who had decided to be sedated palliatively at home. He chose this option over euthanasia because he wanted his body to determine when it would stop living. This is certainly a very bold decision, but technically it is not easy to keep someone permanently sedated using a syringe driver *without influencing life expectancy*. There is always the risk that the patient will develop a tolerance to the drugs and wake up. The dose therefore needs to be constantly adjusted and the distinction between scenarios (a) and (b) becomes very unclear.

In addition, patients under palliative sedation usually do not eat or drink, which also affects their death.

The ethical problems of palliative sedation and its relationship with euthanasia and other end-of-life decisions will be discussed in greater detail later (see p. 137).

8 Psychological support

Although there are no clear boundaries, it is possible to make a distinction between *psychic* symptoms on the one hand, caused by the disease (and the treatment thereof), such as anxiety, depression or confusion, and on the other hand the *psychological* or emotional impact of being seriously ill, such as relationship problems, losing your job, existential issues.

As always, both conditions are treated by traditional healthcare professionals. Psychologists normally play a second-line support role. In many hospitals which have oncology centres, the psychologist from the palliative care team often combines this function with the psycho-oncological care of potentially curable patients.

The added value of a psychologist is, too often, underestimated. This is because healthcare professionals often think their 'intuitive' emotional understanding qualifies them as professionals to deal with such cases. This is partly due to the fact that the term 'psychotherapist' is still not a protected professional title in Belgium. Anyone who has followed an affiliated course on a psychic topic (of a questionable level) for a couple of weekends can add 'therapist' or 'bereavement therapist' or 'psychotherapist' after their name. Of course, some of these people claiming to be therapists are genuine, but there is no guarantee that they will provide professional care to a mentally fragile patient.

Clinical psychology is a profession in its own right, and it requires years of training to be able to deal properly with problems and to act as a second-line reference point.

More than that, it also requires a flexible attitude. Hospital doctors often have a tendency to involve the psychologist indiscriminately. This happens regularly with patients when the doctor has made a mistake, for example by communicating bad news in a particularly awkward manner. The psychologist first has to reassure the patient, and then explain diplomatically (doctors often operate on short fuses) to the doctor how they can tackle the situation better next time.

The psychologist's specific knowledge is essential when crystallising a request for euthanasia. Doctors can make good use of this when there is lack of clarity about depressive moods or the legitimacy of the request. In the same way that a wise doctor will seek advice from a palliative or a medical specialist when their own knowledge in this area is insufficient, they will also seek the opinion of the psychologist in discussions about the patient's end of life.

On 10 March 2008 Minister Laurette Onkelinx presented her National Cancer Plan 2008–2010. Thanks to this initiative, about two hundred and fifty clinical psychologists in Belgium were able to be recruited for oncology departments. In addition, this plan introduced compulsory psychosocial-oncology training for these psychologists. In fact this training was officially recognised by the minister and has been offered for several years by the Cédric Hèle Institute in collaboration with Flemish universities, with great success. The plan also offers communication training for doctors and healthcare professionals (see www.cedric-heleinstituut.be).

9 Social care

People with serious health problems (and their friends and family) often become so overwhelmed that they are no longer able to take care of their material concerns and don't know who or where to ask for help. In an interdisciplinary team, the nurse and the social worker are the perfect people to find the right solutions within the maze of official care facilities, private initiatives, relevant legislation and administrative provisions. They often have to deal with people in crisis: an incurable patient needs a hospital bed installed at their house because they will never walk again; the patient has financial difficulties because they have lost their job; (palliative) leave for the patient's offspring needs to be applied for so that they can look after their parent; the preferred hospice is fully booked and the patient can no longer stay at home alone. The list goes on.

Like the other members of the healthcare system, members of the 'social services' are primarily trained to find solutions and act as 'doers'.

No matter how appealing a particular proposal may appear to the healthcare professional, the patient and their family may disagree completely. The healthcare professional must not take this as a personal affront but must start looking for another alternative without rancour and preferably in conjunction with the patient and/or their family. There are, however, situations in which the patient and even their family are temporarily unable to take certain decisions, and yet a decision has to be made, for example when a patient is forcibly discharged from hospital. In cases such as these, the healthcare professional must take over. It is not easy to strike a balance between being informative (providing information) and being more directive by taking control of a particular facet of the patient's needs. It's a bit like walking a tightrope, and where possible any initiatives taken should be reversible, thereby allowing the patient to make adjustments once they are again capable of doing so. This avoids frustrations and aggressive behaviour, and more importantly guarantees the best possible quality of life. Seriously ill patients have already lost so much control, it is important to involve them in the choice of possible alternatives. This may also help reduce untreatable fear.

This is a task not to be underestimated, requiring significant psychological insight, tact, creativity, flexibility and empathy.

10 Existential suffering and spirituality

People who experience tragic events sometimes come to a literal and figurative standstill and start asking themselves existential questions. In a similar way, patients who are nearing the end of their lives, or with an overwhelming fear of death or separation, are more inclined to ask questions about their existence, about their philosophy of life and their spirituality in relation to the extrasensory world.

A forty-year-old woman with three children and a metastatic cancer may wonder why she was born and why she had children, in short what the meaning of her life has been. A promiscuous thirty-five-year-old gay businessman who is obsessive about safe sex and protection nevertheless discovers that he is HIV positive and in the early stages of AIDS. A sixteen-year-old lovesick adolescent 'dumped' by his sweetheart looks at the canal with suicidal thoughts. A sixty-five-year-old man buys a new car for his retirement but smashes the car to smithereens and becomes completely paralysed, requiring artificial ventilation and feeding.

Many books could be written about these kinds of stories. So long as we are healthy and not facing a crisis or any kind of setback, we tend not to think too long or too hard about the meaning of life, about choices and decisions, or the value of our jobs, and yet throughout humanity, people have endlessly reflected on and written about the inexplicable in an attempt somehow to explain it, to determine whether a single life is part of a greater whole, to contain the collective existential fear of the unknown, the incomprehensible, the meaning of mortality. These reflections led to the birth of different religions – derived from the Latin 'relegere', to reassemble, or 'religare', to connect. The basis of many of these religions is indeed the connection with one or more superhuman, omnipotent, Supreme Being(s). In addition, certain moral values, obligations and rules are adopted collectively. There is nothing wrong with a belief in a supernatural creator if it helps to alleviate existential pain and does not lead to an intolerance of opposing views, which can result in religious wars, torture, beheadings, colonialism, fundamentalist suicide bombers and the rejection of democratic principles. The search for truth is legitimate, but to want to impose and institutionalise a solution or belief is extremely dangerous and damaging.

Liberals, agnostics or atheists tend to base their thinking more on what for them are proven facts, and reject any form of dogmatism. Nevertheless they are no more immune to existential need than anyone else. They just deal with the certainty of uncertainty differently.

The more scientific research provides answers to previously unexplained (natural) phenomena, such as lightning and thunder, the less faith is able to alleviate existential fear. Despite this, many people (often without being true believers) join a religious community and participate in certain rituals such as holy communion, circumcision, ecclesiastical burial. This passive conformist participation is perhaps also related to the fear of being 'ostracised' from the familiar, trusted community life. Not being part of the community requires an active, public stance with the risk of ending up in a new 'uncertainty' which then requires further reflection.

However, the situation may become different when people find themselves in crisis and the masks fall away. Before the existence of effective painkillers, the Christian faith attributed a meaning to physical suffering. This is no longer the case. It is inconceivable today, in our western culture, that an analgesic will be refused for this reason. The same should apply to a request for euthanasia. A population census carried out in Belgium has revealed that more than 80 per cent of Belgians are in favour of the principle. Receptive healthcare professionals confirm that seriously ill patients from Christian communities also ask for euthanasia.

Spiritual pain remains a reality. It differs from individual to individual, depending on cultural, religious and family traditions, and is influenced by each person's own life experience.

Spiritual suffering exacerbates physical symptoms such as pain and psychosocial problems and results in total pain.

Spiritual suffering can be easily missed or ignored. If a patient remarks that they have lost their appetite and is 'therefore losing weight', the doctor or family may respond in a very technical manner by prescribing a diet when in fact it might reflect a profound fear of dying. It is important to be attentive to such details when physical or mental symptoms or social problems turn out to be difficult to resolve. Other comments that should cause concern are:

- I continue to fight bravely (vulnerability);
- no one really understands what I'm going through (isolation);
- my life is worthless (futility);
- why has God forsaken me? (confusion);
- it's my punishment (guilt);
- what can the treatment achieve? (hopelessness);
- I don't want to be a burden (low self-esteem);
- no one cares (sense of abandonment);
- why me? (injustice).

Existential pain may refer to the past, the present and the future.

The past:

- painful memories: shame, feelings of guilt;
- the way a person reflects on their life, their achievements or failures: acceptance or regret;
- the value of their relationships and acquaintances.

The present:

- isolation, anger;
- physical, psychological and social changes;
- increasing dependency;
- the meaning of suffering;
- the meaning of life.

The future:

- fear of death, hopelessness;
- separation anxiety;
- futility.

Dealing with spiritual misery when the patient is nearing the end of their life is one of the most difficult assignments. A listening ear is invaluable. Healthcare professionals must always bear in mind the fact that they have access to the patient's medical history but not their life history, which they can only be told about. Healthcare professionals play a small role in some scenes of the film of the patient's life. These snapshots do not allow the film to be rewritten, but by being an active listener, the professional may be able to change the end of the film. The tragic end is possibly less burdensome if a long-lost son can be persuaded to come and say goodbye. And finally, the support of a religious leader or liberal humanist consultant should not be underestimated, although in our secularised society it is not always easy to get them to the bedside when they are needed. Nevertheless they play an important role in supporting and training healthcare professionals.

11 End-of-life decisions (including euthanasia)

There are many ways to kill. One can stab a knife in your guts; take away your bread; deprive you of the cure for your illness; put you in miserable housing; torture you to death with work; start a war and so on. Most of these methods are not prohibited in our country.

Bertolt Brecht

Euthanasia is just one life-ending decision, and also the least common. Which begs the question: why is it given the most attention by society and the media? The reasons are complex. Firstly because euthanasia is often confused with other 'life-ending' decisions and so is believed to be a regular occurrence, and secondly because there is a general impression that the only time that doctors end the life of a patient is through euthanasia, when in daily practice it happens much more, often under another name.

Even people working in the sector use the word 'euthanasia' to describe completely different situations. In 2000, when it gradually dawned on people that the current Euthanasia Law in Belgium was not such an impossibility, confusion over the various terms led to prosecutions of doctors and nurses working in various Belgian hospitals such as Boom, Asse, Ronse, Namur, Bruges, Edeghem, Liège, Duffel, Veurne, Doornik and Ostend. In other countries where the public debate around euthanasia is quick to ignite, healthcare professionals are accused of performing euthanasia illegally. An example is the recent case in France, when in June 2014 Dr Nicolas Bonnemaison stopped treating patients with medication that no longer provided any benefit to them, and was accused of having euthanised seven patients.

Comments such as 'We must not let the patient suffer; euthanasia is appropriate here for humanitarian reasons', 'The family can't take it any more and asked us to euthanise the patient', 'Euthanasia is dangerous, because we don't want to revert to Hitler-like conditions' are clear examples of how other life-ending decisions are constantly confused with euthanasia.

This confusion is understandable because the term 'euthanasia' over the years has frequently been used and misused to indicate a 'good death'. When a term is used to cover too many different possibilities, it becomes unusable. The word 'euthanasia', however, is well established and will endure because it has media appeal. A newspaper article with the headline: 'Termination of life upon request' will go largely unnoticed, whereas everyone will read an article that begins with 'Euthanasia'.

Before the current law was introduced, 'life-ending treatment' was illegal in Belgium, and indeed a legal definition of the word 'euthanasia' did not exist. People could use it to mean anything they chose (this is still the case in countries without a euthanasia law). The word 'euthanasia' was first introduced in around 1600 by the English philosopher Sir Francis Bacon (1561–1626). He used the term in the literal sense, as derived from Greek: 'eu' ('good'), 'thanatos' ('death'). In fact he meant the ability to die a 'good' death, gently and without pain. In one of his writings he said 'the office of a physician is not only to restore health, but to mitigate pain and dolors; and not only when such mitigation may be conducive to recovery, but also when it may serve to make a fair and easy passage'.

From the meaning thus attributed by Bacon, certain people confused palliative care with (passive) 'euthanasia' (see below). The aim of palliative care, however, is to maximise comfort without any intention of shortening or prolonging the patient's life. Sometimes this may require painkillers or sedatives with unconsciousness, a coma or accelerated death as possible side-effects. Nevertheless the primary intention is pain relief or 'palliative sedation', not the shortening of the patient's life.

Terms such as voluntary, involuntary, passive, active, direct and indirect euthanasia are used. I will not discuss them in depth, because using these outdated terms only adds to the confusion.

Under the impetus of the 1982 reflection in the Netherlands by the Netherlands State Commission on Euthanasia and the Remmelink Commission in 1990, the word 'euthanasia' was given a clear definition. In Belgium, the same clear definition was adopted thanks to the Belgian Advisory Committee on Bioethics. Euthanasia in both countries is defined as 'the deliberate termination of a patient's life by a third party *at the patient's request*'. The third party must be the attending physician.

This definition also helped to clarify what does *not* constitute euthanasia. The following discussion of other life-ending decisions is limited to a practical introduction for those who are interested.

End-of-life decisions

We speak about medical life-ending decisions, although in reality these decisions are not exclusively medical (taken unilaterally by the physician) but also have an ethical component.

From experience and research conducted in most industrialised countries, there are six possible end-of-life decisions that impact on the time of death.

1. Stopping treatment that no longer serves any medical purpose with or without the patient's knowledge/request, for example stopping kidney dialysis of an emaciated terminal kidney patient, or stopping resuscitation.
2. Not starting medically futile treatment, with or without the patient's knowledge/request, such as deciding against follow-up chemotherapy for an incurable cancer patient, or not starting to tube-feed a seriously ill dementia patient.
3. Adjusting the painkiller and/or tranquiliser dosage with or without the patient's knowledge/request, leading to reduced consciousness, coma and even early death in patients such as those with terminal cancer who are suffering unbearable pain. It makes the dying

process easier. When the doctor administers tranquilisers with the express aim of reducing the patient's consciousness it is referred to as palliative sedation.

4. Assisted suicide, such as giving or prescribing a lethal drug that the patient self-administers without the doctor present.

5. Life-ending treatment without the request of the patient, for example a newborn with a severe genetic disorder from which the infant will succumb, possibly after months of agony.

6. Euthanasia. In the three countries with euthanasia laws, it is exclusively restricted to the deliberate termination of a patient's life by a third party at the patient's request.

The current Belgian law only regulates euthanasia, not the five other life-ending decisions.

Comments about these six decisions

Stopping or not starting pointless treatment (1 and 2)

By opting for these 'non-treatment decisions' healthcare professionals renounce 'therapeutic tenacity'. The Belgian Medical Association considers these decisions, together with an increase in painkillers to counter unbearable suffering (3), 'good medical practice'. They are part of a physician's normal professional practice. Of course if the patient is conscious they must be consulted about any of these decisions.

For patients in irreversible comas or those living in persistent vegetative states (PVS), the best approach is to follow the recommendations of the Catholic University of Leuven's Medical Ethics Committee. One in three PVS patients has suffered a heavy skull trauma; one in three has experienced a non-traumatic incident such as a cardiac arrest, and the rest are in the terminal phase of dementia – mostly Alzheimer's. The prognosis for those having suffered a skull trauma is the least gloomy: recovery of cognitive functions is still possible between three and six months after the accident. PVS after oxygen deprivation, however, is very problematic, and after three months you can consider it to be permanent. According to the Catholic University of Leuven's guidelines, all life-support treatment (including the administration of food and fluid) for this last group may be phased out after three months. Each decision is made on an individual basis. In 2005 a media circus and politico-legal battle developed in the USA, and another similar in Italy in 2009, over the life support of two PVS patients, Terri Schiavo and Eluana Englaro respectively. Schiavo lived for 15 years in a vegetative state caused by irrevocable brain damage from oxygen deprivation as a result of a cardiac arrest. Eluana Englaro had been in this state since 1992.

For patients who are no longer able to communicate, the family or close friends should be involved in the decision. This is clearly emphasised in the Belgian Law on Patients' Rights, but unfortunately doesn't happen often enough because of the paternalistic attitude adopted by doctors and their view that 'We know what's best for you'. This belief is also often perpetuated by others: 'Doctor knows best'. However, doctors are often not suitably qualified to communicate this. Lack of knowledge or temporary vulnerability from disease should never be a reason to discontinue efforts to engage in dialogue.

Research carried out by the VUB End-of-life Care Research Group has shown that non-treatment, palliative sedation or increased painkillers due to unbearable suffering occur in about one in two deaths in Europe. About a hundred thousand Belgians die in Belgium annually, which means that approximately fifty thousand deaths per year are medically influenced in some way. As previously mentioned, this is often the result of a unilateral decision. Interestingly, an extensive public debate on this topic has never taken place. Such decisions are almost blindly entrusted to the healthcare professionals. To make mistakes is human and doctors (luckily) are only human. It would be naive to think that among this large number of medically influenced deaths there have been no errors of judgement. The recent debate on euthanasia, on the other hand, has received its fair share of attention. In Belgium it is estimated that euthanasia accounts for approximately one thousand nine hundred deaths per year, all of which are, by definition, carried out in consultation with the patient, since they have to take the initiative.

Previously a decision not to treat a patient was often referred to as 'indirect' or even 'passive' euthanasia. The use of the word 'passive' is confusing because it is difficult to view the disconnection of a breathing machine as 'passive'. If, moreover, the patient in question is in a coma, then clearly the concept of passive euthanasia is a contradiction in terms (the patient is, after all, no longer able to request the euthanasia). In French literature, the term orthothanasia (to die in the right way) is used to describe the decision to forego therapeutic tenacity. This use of the term should be avoided, as it will only lead to more confusion with 'euthanasia'.

Pointless medical treatment or therapeutic tenacity is unacceptable. When a doctor confuses a decision not to treat a patient with euthanasia it can lead to unnecessarily harrowing situations. Consider a patient who has to endure continued dialysis because the doctor refuses to stop 'unless the patient explicitly asks for it', or patients who are not given enough morphine during the dying phase 'because they have not asked for it'. Certain people maintain that these examples illustrate that it was better before the Euthanasia Law was introduced, when in fact these problems are caused by conceptual confusion.

Adjusting painkiller levels (3)

Painkillers/analgesics and/or tranquilisers can also be increased in such a way that the patient no longer has to endure untreatable suffering consciously: this is known as 'palliative sedation'. The aim is to relieve the pain/suffering but it is possible that the increased medication can shorten the patient's life. This was previously incorrectly referred to as 'indirect' or even 'passive' euthanasia. Instead it is a merciful easing of the dying process for a patient who 'will die anyway'. Shortening the patient's life is not the aim, but can be a possible consequence or 'side-effect' of the medication.

Administering significantly higher doses of painkillers and sedatives can also be used as a way to end the patient's life intentionally (see 5 and 6) and not so much to reduce the pain.

Consider the example of a comatose patient in a hospital room being fed potentially deadly products via a tube. A casual passer-by would not be able to determine whether the purpose of the medication is to relieve pain (3) resulting in a coma, or intentionally to end the patient's life unrequested (5) or euthanasia (6). The distinction between pain control during the fight against death, the intentional ending of a patient's life without them having requested it (possibly at the request of the family) and euthanasia is razor thin and therefore often thought of as a 'twilight zone'.

This means that doctors are in a position to 'help' patients end their lives without facing any consequences. Once the patient is dead it is very difficult for an outsider to determine the doctor's exact intention when administering the medication: whether it was mercy, the intentional shortening of the patient's life, or euthanasia. Before the introduction of the Euthanasia Law, the only non-punishable intention for doctors was 'mercy pain relief' or 'acting in an emergency'. Euthanasia was not allowed, and ending a patient's life without request was unmentionable, which added yet another reason (for doctors) to operate secretively, without consultation, and to not use the right process. Thanks to the law, the doctor is now required to consult with the patient and the family to avoid the above-mentioned allegations.

Palliative sedation is often offered as an alternative to euthanasia. The patient is induced into a coma so that they are no longer conscious of any symptoms, and they 'spontaneously die' from their illness. There is nothing wrong with this if it is the patient's choice. The reality of the twilight zone is that it is never clear whether palliative sedation was necessary for a given patient. In some cases, the doctor has no choice but to take a unilateral decision; it is unthinkable that a doctor would not administer some form of pain relief to a demented patient who is crying out in pain from bedsores. Nevertheless, for as long as the patient is in a fit state, their views must be consulted where possible. Failing this, the family must be notified. In addition, during sedation either the administration of food and fluid is often stopped on the grounds that nutrition is no longer needed because the patient will die anyway, or the dosages of sedatives are increased in order to 'speed up' death. This fosters the belief that palliative sedation allows the doctor the sovereign right to end a patient's life under another name.

In 2013 Livia Anquinet, in her doctoral dissertation, reported that the incidence of deaths due to palliative sedation had roughly doubled since the introduction of the Belgian Euthanasia Law, from 8 per cent (eight thousand out of a hundred thousand) to 15 per cent (fifteen thousand). This disturbing increase is undoubtedly due to doctors being more empathetic to the suffering of terminal patients, but it may also be due to unapproved euthanasia requests. In addition, the incidence of palliative sedation is twice as high in French-speaking Belgium as in Flanders, whereas incidences of registered euthanasia are six times lower. This is probably due to cultural differences between the North and the South of Belgium; French-speaking doctors tend to be more paternalistic towards their patients than Flemish doctors. In the UK the number of palliative sedations is higher still, around 18 per cent.

Sixty-year-old Marcel Engelborghs, a flamboyant alderman in Tongres, was terminally ill and knew that he wanted a self-imposed death before the decline became intolerable for him. He went public with his decision because he wanted to break the prevailing taboo around euthanasia, but then panicked when initially prescribed palliative sedation instead because, according to his medical team, he was not yet 'terminal'. Ultimately, however, he was euthanised at the Catholic University Hospital, Leuven on 5 March 2008, possibly as a result of the widespread media attention which he himself had created.

Many patients fail to appreciate the distinction between euthanasia and palliative sedation, both of which put an end to unbearable suffering. Out of respect for patients' rights, both options should be discussed with a patient who wishes to be relieved of their pain. Some patients, given the option of palliative sedation, ask (aloud) what the point is of lying unconscious for days or weeks before dying.

And in conclusion, palliative care is a good alternative when therapeutic tenacity is waived, which is why palliative care is sometimes even equated to 'passive euthanasia'. The late Queen Fabiola even asked me once to explain the difference between palliative care and euthanasia (see p. 21).

Assisted suicide (4)

In an assisted suicide the doctor provides assistance to a person who wants to commit suicide by giving them a prescription or by providing them with lethal drugs. The doctor then leaves the patient to end their life at the moment of their choosing *without the doctor present*. A commonly held perception is that with assisted suicide the lethal drugs are placed by the doctor on the patient's bedside table, whereas with euthanasia they are placed on the patient's tongue.

In Belgium, assisted suicide should not be confused with euthanasia. Euthanasia is not restricted to the doctor giving a lethal injection. It can take the form of a lethal drink which the patient administers themselves. In contrast to assisted suicide, however, the doctor remains available for the patient, stays in the room and accepts the medical responsibility. For instance, if the patient is about to awake from a coma, the doctor will put an end to the patient's life with an injection. There is no specification in the Euthanasia Law as to the manner in which the patient's life should be terminated. It is therefore quite possible, in Belgium, that the patient can administer the lethal medication themselves, in the presence of the doctor. However, in practice this rarely happens.

Life-ending treatment not at the request of the patient (5)

Such treatment is common among doctors who measure the quality of life according to their own standards: 'If I was in their shoes, I wouldn't want to live'. Previously it was referred to as 'involuntary' or 'unsolicited' euthanasia.

As already mentioned, it is difficult to determine accurately the doctor's intention in 'sedating a patient to death'. It appears that some doctors still struggle with the idea of terminating a person's life without it having been requested. A 'lethal drip' is concocted in such a way that the patient will die only after three days. The doctor responsible can tell themselves – and friends and family – that their intention was palliative sedation (3), thereby negating the fact that their original intention was life termination.

It is also possible that the original intention was palliative sedation, but that after a few days or weeks, possibly under pressure from the exhausted family, the doctor may change their mind and increase the doses to accelerate death (see p. 125). But for the outside world it remains 'palliative sedation'. In this way the Euthanasia Law is very neatly sidestepped and the doctor has not performed 'euthanasia' since this was 'not a case of euthanasia'.

The lives of seriously ill newborn babies and young minors without the mental capacity to ask for euthanasia may also be terminated without request (see p. 194).

From the previously quoted research at the VUB, it appears that prior to the introduction of the Euthanasia Law, Flemish doctors ended lives without the patient's knowledge up to four times more than Dutch doctors. Since the law was introduced, the number of unrequested life terminations in Belgium has halved, a further illustration that the current law has not resulted in misuse.

Euthanasia (6)

Euthanasia therefore refers exclusively to the 'deliberate termination of a person's life by a doctor *at the explicit and repeated request of the patient* who is desperate due to unbearable suffering', previously also known as 'direct', 'voluntary' and 'active' euthanasia.

For the sake of clarity, the adjectives have been omitted. It is very important to use the correct terminology, especially, for example, when considering France's so-called Euthanasia Law. Since the recent introduction of the Leonetti Law in France, it is now possible to refuse treatment even if the life is shortened as a result. As the French themselves cynically maintain they can now be passively 'allowed to die'. In Belgium this falls under the 'non-treatment decisions' (1 and 2) and is explicitly included in the Belgian Patients' Rights Law. The active injection of a lethal product on request – euthanasia – is still illegal in France. Think of the drama of Chantal Sébire, a teacher with a gruesome facial tumour, who in 2008 pleaded with the then president to be euthanised, to no avail. She ultimately committed suicide.

The following example tries to illustrate that in a society with access to cutting-edge medical technology, the distinction between passive and active treatment is outdated and, at the same time, absurd. Consider, for example, a patient who is completely paralysed being kept alive by a ventilator and feeding tube. This patient is in a medically hopeless situation, is suffering unbearably and asks to be euthanised. In Belgium, the doctor is allowed to carry out this request provided certain criteria are respected. Because the law does not specify exactly how the euthanasia must be performed, the doctor, *in this specific instance*, is left with five methods to choose from:

1. They take a gun and shoot the patient.
2. They close the vent of the breathing apparatus (ventilator); the patient suffocates and dies.
3. They sedate the patient first and then close the ventilator.
4. They stop the artificial feeding and fluid administration, causing the patient to die after about two weeks.
5. They inject a lethal substance into the patient's vein.

Methods 1, 2 and 4 are objectionable. According to 'old' reasoning methods 2 and 4 would be classified as a *passive* intervention. In contrast, method 5 would be classified as *active* intervention.

This example illustrates that cutting off a patient's artificial ventilation is as active a treatment as administering a lethal injection. The intention in both instances is the same – to end the patient's life upon request – the only difference is the technique. For some there may be a psychological difference.

The current Belgian Euthanasia Law has helped stimulate the debate around all end-of-life decisions as well as offering legal certainty to the doctor, the patient and their family.

The public debate in the next few years will undoubtedly be about all the other end-of-life decisions; those which are considered 'good medical practice' where decisions are still, too often, taken without consulting the patient.

12 Belgian euthanasia (law) in practice

What is the benefit of laws without morals?

Horatius

The desirability of a legal framework to regulate euthanasia has been covered in many excellent books and papers (see also the situation in Belgium in the table below). In this chapter I will limit the discussion to practical considerations, stemming from after the law became a reality.

And yet there are still those, primarily from countries which do not have a euthanasia law, who argue that a legal framework would lead to abuse. This is absurd. If we extrapolate this logic to other laws and regulations, then all legislation should be abolished. Traffic regulations stipulate that a green light means go and a red light means stop. This is a necessary social standard. And just as the rules of the road do not guarantee that there won't be any infringements, so the Euthanasia Law does not. However, since its introduction it has become clear that the Euthanasia Law has not led to any abuse. In addition, thanks to the law, there has been a significant reduction (around 50 per cent) in the incidence of unrequested life-ending treatment (a practice that is very difficult to monitor). Finally, no one is required, as a result of the law, to request or apply euthanasia; it is voluntary.

The need for a Euthanasia Law

The Belgian Euthanasia Law has been in force since 2002. But even before then, euthanasia was practiced, despite the fact that Belgium has, for years, benefited from excellent palliative care (palliative care was developed in Belgium before the euthanasia debate took place, whereas in the Netherlands it was the other way round: developments in palliative care came after the Euthanasia Law had been voted in). Palliative care can alleviate much, but not all, terminal suffering. In such instances, it occurred that an empathetic doctor could choose to end a dying patient's life to relieve their suffering.

This is known as mercy killing. The doctor reacts in an emergency situation in which they have to choose between two potentially conflicting values: to end someone's suffering and to try and save their life. There are times when the only way to end a person's suffering is to end their life. As previously mentioned, it is called 'euthanasia' when the termination of the patient's life is performed at their request; when it happens without their knowledge it is referred to as life termination without request. Before the Euthanasia Law was introduced both of these practices were commonplace, although not acknowledged, because doctors did not want to be held accountable before a judge. Assuming that protecting a patient's life is considered morally superior to ending the patient's suffering, the doctor could be accused of manslaughter at the very least. Few doctors were willing to run this risk, and many suffering patients were left out in the cold as a result. Moreover, because these activities were not transparent and often done without consultation, the term 'euthanasia' was not defined very accurately. At the time, the term was also used for mercy killing without the patients' knowledge, as still happens today in countries without a euthanasia law.

Spokesmen of the Christian Democrats, in particular, were of the view that the legal concept of the 'emergency situation' was sufficiently protective. They felt that doctors who performed these mercy killings did so out of *pity and compassion*, and only once all attempts at (palliative) care had failed. They claimed that these situations of 'acute emergency' were extremely exceptional, and that there was therefore no need for a change in the law.

Meanwhile, the reality clearly demonstrated that, despite good palliative care, terminal suffering is not at all exceptional. Even opponents of the Euthanasia Law who had previously claimed that requests for euthanasia were very rare had to acknowledge that this was so. Ironically they are now requesting more resources in order to deal with all these requests for euthanasia in a caring and professional manner. One can't help wondering how these former opponents responded to such requests before the law was introduced.

These politicians also overlooked the fact that unbearable suffering is also possible for patients not in a terminal phase and beyond the need for palliative care, for example in patients with terrible neurological disorders, paralysis, loss of bodily functions, etc. Cases such as these cannot be considered as *mercy killing out of pity and compassion* but rather life termination at the request of non-terminal, yet suffering, patients, out of deep *empathy and respect* for their *right to self-determination*. Given that certain principled Christians find this last principle unacceptable, they preferred to stick with the precedence of 'an emergency' without a legal framework.

There was therefore a need for a democratically chosen law to protect doctors against the random 'emergency situation' case and to give seriously ill patients (both terminal and non-terminal) the right to request euthanasia. In addition, the law needed to provide a very clear definition of the term 'euthanasia' to allow for transparency of treatment that hitherto took place in the 'twilight zone' (see p. 127). Ultimately the law was necessary because according to Article 394 of the Belgian Penal Code 'premeditated killing' is murder. This is true even if the person concerned – the patient – has given their consent.

Although the Euthanasia Law is becoming more known (thanks in part to public testimonials such as that of Belgian Nobel Laureate Christian De Duve, who chose euthanasia), the general public, doctors and other healthcare professionals are still not familiar enough with it.

It is a patient-friendly law that gives seriously ill patients the *right to ask* for their lives to be ended, which is not the same as an unconditional *right to euthanasia*.

And doctors maintain the right to refuse any given request.

The Belgian Euthanasia Law in a nutshell

As a result of the Euthanasia Law, life termination by request is no longer prosecutable, provided certain conditions are met.

Conditions and procedure

Euthanasia should only be carried out by a doctor. According to the Euthanasia Law of 2002 the applicant must be at least 18 years of age – and be 'capable of discernment'. They should be aware of their situation and be informed of any remaining treatment options and their prognoses. Patients need to be diagnosed with a 'medically hopeless', serious, incurable condition as a result of disease or accident (for example paralysis), which is causing them 'unbearable suffering'. The affliction may be physical (for example cancer) or psychiatric (for example bipolar disorder). Psychiatric patients should of course be capable of discernment. The medical hopelessness – the incurable aspect – is determined by the physician. The unbearable suffering – the human hopelessness – is determined by the patient themselves (as already mentioned, the suffering must be caused by an incurable condition). The patient has to win the doctor's empathy by convincing them of their suffering. Much was written about medical hopelessness and unbearable suffering in 2009 following the request for euthanasia from 93-year-old Amélie Van Esbeen who claimed to be suffering from 'life fatigue' (see box).

The patient must request euthanasia 'voluntarily, repeatedly and continually'. The request must also be made in writing. It can be done on any piece of paper and should at least contain the words 'I want euthanasia', the date of the request, as well as the applicant's name and signature. If the patient for some reason is no longer able to do this for themselves (paralysis for example) then someone else can write it for them under certain conditions.

Life fatigue

In March 2009 the Belgian media was full of reports about Amélie Van Esbeen's request for euthanasia due to 'life fatigue'. Does someone who is quite simply 'tired of life' have the right to euthanasia? Or how serious must an incurable condition be before euthanasia is accorded? The subject has already been debated in the Netherlands, notably during the trial of Philip Sutorius, a general practitioner who helped Edward Brongersma to die. The elderly man had no serious medical condition but was suffering unbearably from a 'life fatigue'. As a result, it was concluded that the cause of the unbearable suffering was not important. It is too simplistic to limit suffering to incurable physical or psychiatric conditions. Pain and suffering are sensations generated in the brain. All suffering, even without clearly identifiable causes, is therefore psychic and existential. This reasoning, however, doesn't help with a euthanasia request due to 'life fatigue'. There is no group of persons qualified to judge whether someone is irrevocably without hope, has had enough of life and is suffering unbearably and therefore can be euthanised.

In the case of Amelie Van Esbeen, it initially sounded as if her request for euthanasia was prompted because she was tired of life. Later it became apparent that it was as a result of various ailments. She was losing her sight, she had problems with her hearing, she was bedridden and had limited independence. Individually these ailments may be bearable but together they form an unbearable incurable condition also known as poly-pathology.

Edward Brongersma and Amelie Van Esbeen's stories show many similarities. Both of them requested euthanasia because of the hopelessness of their suffering.

In the same way that palliative care will never eliminate all requests for euthanasia, neither will the best possible supportive care for elderly people provide the answer to all existential pain. It calls for a public debate.

Amelie Van Esbeen died by euthanasia on 1 April 2009.

In addition, the attendant doctor must discuss the case with 'a colleague' who has examined the patient's file and who must offer formal, though non-binding, 'written advice'. This serves two purposes. It provides the patient with confirmation of the hopelessness of their medical condition, as well as providing support for the doctor.

In parallel with this, the attendant doctor must complete a certain procedure. This is to ensure that all euthanasia requests are handled with care. The physician must inform the patient (in language that they understand) of their state of health and life expectancy. The physician must also discuss all remaining treatment and palliative-care options (and their side-effects), without enforcing these options on the patient.

The attendant doctor must then discuss the request with the nursing staff involved in the patient's healthcare and the patient's family – but only with the patient's permission. This ensures that the patient is able – for whatever reason – to conceal their desire for euthanasia from certain family members. This is a fundamental patient right that also applies to all medical procedures.

Euthanasia in prison: what about mentally ill persons held in prison?

In principle, mentally ill patients – and other prisoners – have the right to request euthanasia. In fact, euthanasia has already been carried out on a prisoner suffering from terminal cancer.

The issue of psychiatric patients held in prison is more complex. In Dirk Leestmans's sensational *Panorama* broadcast at the end of 2013 (for which the entire *Panorama* team was awarded the League of Human Rights prize) he discusses the request for euthanasia made by Frank Van den Bleeken. Frank Van den Bleeken is regarded as an incurable psychiatric patient but has been in prison for almost thirty years without any significant psychiatric treatment. In the Netherlands, the Pompe Stichting (Pompe Foundation) offers customised palliative psychiatric treatment, and the patient agreed to follow it. As a result, the euthanasia question was suspended. Moreover, it is also not clear whether his request for euthanasia is due to unbearable suffering caused by the psychiatric illness, or by the hopeless context of the prison. Frank Van den Bleeken appealed against the Belgian state because his request for transfer to the Netherlands was refused, and he submitted a new request for euthanasia. In September 2014 Frank Van den Bleeken was finally granted permission to be transferred to a hospital to honour his euthanasia request. He was due to have been euthanised on 11 January 2015 in the medical department of the prison in Bruges, because no hospital was found willing to admit him. However, at the very last moment, Dr Marc Cosyns, the treating physician, drew back for unknown reasons.

Euthanasia for non-terminal patients: the deaf-mute twins and the transgender

Mario Verstraete, the first officially euthanised patient in Belgium, was not in the final stages of a terminal illness, and it seems that euthanasia of non-terminal patients provokes uproar – certainly in the foreign press. And yet since the introduction of the Euthanasia Law in 2002, 6–13 per cent of registered euthanasia cases are for non-terminal patients. In the 2014 report (covering 2012–2013) by the Federal Euthanasia Commission, 433 (including 120 patients with neuropsychiatric disorders) out of a total of 3239 euthanised patients were not in the final stages of a terminal illness (13 per cent). The legislature has rightly recognised that unbearable suffering is possible as a result of a serious, incurable non-terminal disease (see p. 150). The difference between terminal and non-terminal is not always clear (see p. 166). Two cases that made headlines in 2013 seemed to capture the public's imagination in such a way as to spark highly emotional reactions, from people who had no prior knowledge about the cases in question. Among the things said about the deaf-mute twins Marc and Eddy Verbessem, who were threatened by blindness, was that they needed a better environment and better care. In reality they were perfectly surrounded by their family and the community, in which they were able to live independently. The threat of losing their sight and independence made their request for euthanasia extremely compelling. In addition, both twins also had other unbearable physical suffering. They were Catholic and had the last rites administered by a priest before they died.

The case of transgender Nathan Verhelst was reduced, in most (foreign) media, to an identity crisis as a result of failed surgery. Without violating professional confidentiality, it can be stated that in reality Nathan Verhelst was not only living with mental anguish but also physically unbearable suffering as a result of an incurable combined physical and psychiatric condition. Had the patient not been transgender, his euthanasia would not have attracted so much press attention.

These two cases do not, obviously, mean that all deaf and dumb patients who are going blind will request euthanasia, nor that all patients who have had failed transgender surgery automatically qualify for euthanasia. Every request for euthanasia must be examined individually and all factors carefully weighed up. The twins with the support of their local doctor, David Dufour, took two years to find a medical institution prepared to perform the euthanasia. Nathan Verhelst was treated by the UL team (see p. 167) for 20 months before the euthanasia was performed.

The above also applies to the elderly couple from Meerbeke near Brussels who in 2011 requested to be euthanised together. The 83-year-old husband had terminal prostate cancer, whereas his 78-year-old-wife was suffering from various non-terminal old-age ailments – poly-pathology. Both situations were reviewed separately and approved. In this situation, it would have been inhumane not to allow both procedures to take place simultaneously.

The above examples are the exceptions and not representative of the thousands of approved requests from terminally ill cancer patients. They are unfortunately repeated over and over again in countries where a euthanasia law is being debated, and exploited by opponents to illustrate the extent to which ethical end-of-life treatment in Belgium has been 'derailed'.

If the above is all in order, the euthanasia may be performed on the same day that the written request is signed by a terminally ill patient.

Euthanasia can also be performed even when the patient is not expected to die in the foreseeable future (non-terminally ill) as was the case with Mario Verstraete, suffering from multiple sclerosis, the first person to use the Euthanasia Law. His story was the subject of Nic Balthazar's beautiful 2012 movie *Tot altijd* (*Until Forever*). In such instances, a third doctor – a psychiatrist or a specialist of the given condition – must be consulted and a waiting period of at least one month has to be respected after the date of the written request (see p. 168).

An anticipated declaration for euthanasia

Patients in Belgium can specify in an 'anticipated declaration for euthanasia' that a doctor should apply euthanasia if they fall into an irreversible coma. A model of this declaration of intent can be found in the LEIF brochure (see p. 161) or on the internet. It is valid for a maximum of five years and must be renewed at the end of this period.

The declaration

After euthanasia is carried out, the doctor is required to fill out a registration document and send it within four working days by registered post to the Belgian Federal Euthanasia Control and Evaluation Commission (Federal Euthanasia Commission). The Commission then checks that the legal conditions and procedures were complied with and must deliver its opinion within two months. In this manner, the Commission members act as a buffer between the medical field and the judicial authorities. They assess whether the spirit rather than the letter of the law was respected: is the patient a person capable of discernment, in a medically hopeless situation experiencing unbearable suffering who has voluntarily and repeatedly requested euthanasia? If so, the Commission then has the power to approve the 'global' declaration, even if there have been procedural errors. A doctor who was dismissed in early 2003 from a large hospital in Asse was subsequently cleared in June 2005.

The Commission had approved the declaration in question in 2003 despite the absence of a written request. The file provided sufficient proof that the request was made voluntarily by the patient.

The Belgian Euthanasia Law extended to include minors capable of discernment

In February 2014 the Belgian law was extended to include minors with a 'capacity for discernment'. The main reasons for adopting the amendment to the law are summarised below:

- Suffering is not restricted to a certain age. This discrimination was already noted and published years ago by the Belgian Medical Association. Similar recommendations for a legislative initiative were recently published by the Belgian Royal Academy of Medicine.

- Euthanasia of minors is not new; it has been practised for years in the same way that adults were euthanised long before the Euthanasia Law was introduced. It is a deeply unpleasant experience for everyone concerned: the patient, the family members who don't have the opportunity of a proper mourning process, and for the doctor, whose only legal defence is the 'emergency situation', a fairly precarious defence. As a result, few doctors were willing to do this and would rather opt for palliative sedation. The number of (terminal) palliative sedations doubled since the introduction of the Euthanasia Law in 2002 (8 per cent of all deaths before 2002, currently 15 per cent). Terminal sedation could be administered at the request of the patient, or even without their request, which again puts the doctor in the spotlight. No compulsory declaration for the Commission is required, as is the case with euthanasia – a practice that has never been questioned by opponents of the Euthanasia Law.

- No-one is required by law either to perform or request euthanasia. The highly emotional media response to euthanasia was caused by a broader definition of euthanasia in countries such as the UK, the USA and Canada: the concept of euthanasia in these countries covers both the deliberate termination of life 'at the request of the patient' and 'without their request', as in terminal sedation (see above).

- According to the Belgian Law on Patients' Rights (2002) a minor of any age, with the capacity of discernment, can refuse treatment (even if it will save their life). This is binding and has never been contested.

According to the amended law, any minor 'capable of discernment' with unbearable *physical* suffering as a result of a *terminal condition* may request euthanasia. The capacity for discernment must be formally confirmed by a psychologist or child psychiatrist. In addition, the parents have to give their consent. This has been possible in the Netherlands since 2002 for children aged 12 and above with the permission of their parents. Once the children reach the age of 16, the parents just need to be informed. In such cases, the capacity for discernment needs to be confirmed by the attendant doctor. The problem with incapacitated minors, such as newborns, who by definition are unable to request euthanasia, is discussed under the 'Groningen protocol' (see p. 194).

Why are willing doctors still hard to find?

Many doctors feel uncomfortable when they are faced with dying or decisions about ending a patient's life. This is largely due to their training which focuses almost exclusively on healing. Future doctors are trained to be able to talk about all symptoms and possible treatments of the rarest of diseases which they are unlikely ever to encounter, and yet in most medical schools, very little attention is paid to the most common human 'ailment' (dying) and all that goes with it.

It is difficult for doctors, after completing their studies, to acquire extensive experience in terminal care. A GP treats fewer than five dying patients a year on average, which amounts to two hundred deaths during a career of forty years. This is one of the arguments in favour of having specialist palliative teams and units available to provide support for the doctor in complex clinical or psychosocial situations.

According to the reports of the Federal Euthanasia Commission euthanasia is applied in only 2 per cent of all deaths. Any given doctor will therefore only be confronted with a request for euthanasia a few times in their life (even taking into account requests that are refused). Although the Belgian Euthanasia Law provides for the mandatory consultation of a second doctor (and a third doctor in cases of non-terminal patients), even these doctors have limited experience in this area. For this reason, as in the Netherlands, a doctors' forum has been established to provide training on these specific issues.

There are other reasons why doctors are unwilling to perform euthanasia:

- For some, there is still the fear of control or persecution. Doctors are trained to be independent, autonomous decision-makers and not involved in social control. However, they are now legally able to do what was previously done in secret. The registration document which is sent to the Federal Euthanasia Commission protects them against third-party interpretation of their intentions.

- The fact that there are sufficient other unilateral ways (around 50 per cent) to end a patient's life *where the doctor's intention can never really be known*: for example, stopping or not starting treatment or the unilaterally decided increase in painkillers leading to unconsciousness, coma and possible death.

- Institutional influence or social pressure still plays an important role. Doctors in some hospitals or residential care centres ultimately give in to the 'anti-euthanasia' climate of the institution. The influence can be subtle: the realisation that a contract extension depends on it or that it reduces the chances of promotion. Certain GPs are afraid that they will be labelled 'Dr Death' in their area and might lose patients as a result.

- No medical indication yet. Some doctors may feel that patients at a certain stage of a condition are not yet eligible for euthanasia.

- Doctors can refuse for ideological or ethical reasons. It is easier for doctors who, through their belief systems, are able to offer euthanasia as an equivalent alternative than for their colleagues who are as yet unable to do so. The former can discuss all possible options with the patient in a calm, open way. It is every patient's democratic right to be informed of all options by healthcare professionals. Doctors who do not want to practice euthanasia – which is, of course, their right – should be obliged to refer these patients to a fellow doctor. A patient who has requested euthanasia cannot be helped by a doctor who is having a crisis of conscience. Unfortunately, some healthcare professionals who, prior to the introduction of the Euthanasia Law, saw palliative care as the only solution are now playing catch-up to be able to include 'euthanasia' in their portfolio. There is nothing wrong with this per se, unless it is an attempt to redirect requests for euthanasia and revert to 'palliative obstinacy', a problem of not being able to let go, of thinking that there are still other options available. But these physicians are making the same mistake as doctors who do not want to refer their patients to palliative teams and insist on 'therapeutic persistence.

- Another not insignificant reason why doctors struggle with euthanasia is not so much ideological as because in these instances the patient is in charge and is able to set the tone and take the initiative. Many doctors do not know how to deal with this. Doctors are frequently still trained to adopt a paternalistic attitude towards their patients, to think for them, or to jokingly remark that doctors don't like patients who take the initiative. As already mentioned, this is one of the important spin-offs of the Euthanasia Law: patients are now officially aware that they themselves can take the initiative and would like to see this extended to the entire illness process and not only at the end of their lives.

- A number of doctors connected to palliative teams or units struggled, particularly when the Euthanasia Law was initially introduced, with simultaneously performing the roles of palliative and euthanasia doctor. This is understandable. These doctors fought for years to get palliative care recognised by both their peers and patients and feared, albeit without cause, that their efforts would be nullified. It also gave rise to ludicrous situations where doctors would not perform euthanasia while working as palliative doctors but were available to do so 'after hours'.

- And finally, uncertainty and lack of experience play a very important role. This was the reason for establishing the LEIF doctors' forum.

What is LEIF?

The main reason why some doctors are still hesitant when confronted with a request for euthanasia is a lack of knowledge, experience and a sense of uncertainty. If they seek advice or support from colleagues – a second or third doctor – not only is that hard to find but these colleagues are often equally uncertain and also lack experience in this area.

A similar situation was experienced in the Netherlands, despite years of tolerant policies and the registration of euthanasia practice since 1990. The Koninklijke Nederlandsche Maatschappij ter bevordering van de Geneeskunst – KNMG (Royal Dutch Society for the Promotion of Medicine), the Dutch equivalent of the Belgian Medical Association, took the initiative at the end of the nineties to set up a specialist group of doctors (GPs). They were given intensive training in providing 'expert' and independent second opinions about euthanasia requests. The group known as SCEN (Steun en Consultatie Euthanasie Nederland, Netherlands Euthanasia Support and Consultation) currently boasts more than six hundred members. A recent analysis has clearly demonstrated the added value provided by these doctors and advises countries wanting to introduce a euthanasia law to establish a similar network of doctors in conjunction with it.

I took a similar initiative in Flanders some months after the Euthanasia Law entered into force, which resulted in the LevensEinde Informatie Forum (LEIF, Life's End Information Forum) being established. This forum is an open initiative supported by people and societies that aspire to a dignified death for everyone, where respect for the patient's will is paramount. The so-called LEIF doctors are trained through this forum to fulfil a similar function to that of the SCEN doctors. The forum unites more than four hundred LEIF doctors (GPs and hospital doctors) from Flanders and Brussels. They follow training on euthanasia, decisions that need to be taken at the end of one's life and palliative care options in Flanders. In this way, colleagues learn from each other.

LEIF doctors support their colleagues in different ways:

- communicative: how to respond to a given question; how to deal with family and other concerned parties;

- content: is it about a 'real question' or rather about a need for pain relief, palliative care, palliative sedation or there is talk of therapeutic obstinacy?
- medico-technical: how to perform euthanasia carefully;
- legal: for example how to complete the registration document.

In contrast to SCEN doctors, consultation among LEIF doctors is not restricted to advice about euthanasia. LEIF doctors may also be consulted on all end-of-life decisions as well as palliative-care options.

LEIF doctors provide support and advice for euthanasia requests but generally do not perform the euthanasia and shouldn't be considered as travelling 'Dr Deaths'. Many LEIF doctors also give lectures on end-of-life concerns, when asked.

In addition to LEIF doctors, there are other doctors (in palliative teams for example) with sufficient expertise to assist their colleagues competently with end-of-life issues. Many palliative doctors have also joined the LEIF doctors' forum.

Yanna Van Wesemael, who conducted a thorough analysis of the work done by LEIF doctors for her PhD, came to similar conclusions in the defence of her thesis at the end of 2011.

Consulting a LEIF doctor has one advantage: you can be sure that they will agree with the principle of euthanasia. The Federal Euthanasia Commission suggested in its first report that the impact of LEIF doctors may at least partly explain why more than 80 per cent of the euthanasia declarations in Belgium come from Flanders and only 20 per cent from Wallonia (the French-speaking part of Belgium containing 40 per cent of the Belgian population).

With the support of the Flemish Government a LEIF helpline was established. Following the acquittal of nurse Els Op de Weerdt, who was accused of murdering her aunt, LEIF introduced end-of-life training for nurses in 2006. These LEIF nurses may act as points of reference in the workplace for their fellow nurses. Since 2008 LEIF also provides training for other professionals such as psychologists, physiotherapists, pharmacists, religious leader, liberal humanist consultants, social workers etc. In this way it is hoped that end-of-life decisions will become more transparent, not only for the relevant healthcare professionals, but also other professions. When I was asked by a criminal lawyer, Jef Vermassen, to act as an expert for the defence during the Els Op de Weerdt trial, certain parliamentarians demanded that I resign as Chairman of the Federal Euthanasia Commission as 'the Chairman should not testify in favour of an illegally performed euthanasia'. What Els Op de Weerdt did – admittedly not in the best way – had absolutely nothing to do with euthanasia, but was a perfect example of a case of mercy killing (see p. 171): her aunt was on the ward where Els was on night duty and was howling with pain as she was dying. With no doctor contactable, Els took the initiative of injecting her with a large dose of morphine.

Since 2008, LEIF has published the LEIF brochure, which is available to the public and can be obtained in libraries, pharmacies and local administrative offices. The aim of this brochure is to clarify the legal options available to patients at the end of their lives: their patient's rights, palliative care and euthanasia.

In addition, the LEIF brochure contains all legal and ready-to-use declaration forms to allow patients to determine the circumstances of their own deaths in a timely manner and to plan the requisite care. These include the advance 'negative' declaration of intent (living will), the advance euthanasia declaration of intent, an organ donation declaration of intent and a burial mode declaration. More than four hundred thousand copies have been distributed over the past six years, showing the extent of the need for information about the end of life. The LEIF brochure and the legal forms can also be downloaded from www.leif.be. Completing declarations of intent is not restricted to the end of life, and can even save lives. Since Marieke Vervoort, with her 'papers in order', won gold and silver medals at the Paralympic Games in 2012 in London, she has found a new lease of life, and her original request for euthanasia has been dropped. She is in full training for the next Paralympic Games in Rio de Janeiro in 2016. Nevertheless, knowing that she can pull the emergency brake at any given moment has given her peace of mind.

The LEIF card was introduced in February 2013. It resembles a plastic bank card and contains information about which declarations the owner has signed and the name of a contact person. It fits easily in a person's wallet. The first LEIF card was formally given to Professor Etienne Vermeersch, philosopher and ethicist at the University of Ghent, because he was the first to introduce euthanasia as a debatable subject on television in 1971. In just a few months, more than fifteen thousand LEIF cards were requested.

LEIF, in the eyes of many who are opposed to euthanasia (but clearly do not oppose intellectual dishonesty), remains an organisation that promotes euthanasia. The truth is that LEIF and associated partners only consider euthanasia as one option at the end of life, in the same way as other life-ending decisions and palliative care. LEIF wants to be able to discuss all possible options for a dignified end of life and inform the patient in a neutral way.

In summer 2010 the first French-speaking LEIF doctors, médecins EOL (End-of-Life Doctors) received their training and now, along with their Flemish colleagues, fall under a federal umbrella.

For years, opponents of euthanasia tried all possible means to prevent LEIF doctors from being remunerated for their expertise and opinion in assessing euthanasia requests, each of which takes about three to four hours. They even submitted a request to the Council of State to annul the Royal Decree regulating these payments. In December 2014, the Council of State decided to reject this request. LEIF doctors are now paid about €150 per consultation. In the Netherlands, SCEN doctors have received a fee of €330 per consultation since the introduction of the Dutch Euthanasia Law (2002).

In order to make LEIF more accessible to the general public, LEIF West Flanders was founded in Bruges in early 2013 at the instigation of André Van Nieuwkerke and Dr Luc Proot. A similar initiative was taken by Jacinta De Roeck in Antwerp. There is currently a base in Brussels, Ghent and Oudenaarde, and other LEIF points will follow.

Also in 2013, LEIF launched, together with the deMens.nu 'Waardig Levenseinde' (Dignified Life's End) Chair at the VUB, the Palliative Care Forum, Omega and Topaz and partners, intensive training in palliative care, and PALM training, intended for medical doctors and masters.

And finally, at the end of 2013, LEIF celebrated its tenth anniversary with a symposium at the Royal Flemish Theatre in Brussels. During the celebrations, the first LEIFtime Achievement Award – a bronze sculpture created by the famous Flemish artist Willy Peeters – was deservedly awarded to the three feisty honorary senators who established the current Euthanasia Law: Jeannine Leduc, Myriam Vanlerberghe and Jacinta De Roeck.

How to respond to a request for euthanasia

When confronted directly or indirectly with a request for euthanasia it should always be taken seriously and an attempt made to ascertain whether it is a 'pseudo-question' or a genuine request. Pseudo-questions often mask other questions. In most cases they are a cry for help for better psychological, medical or palliative care – 'Please put an end to this pain, I can't take it any more' – which can be met, at least temporarily, by harnessing the right, tailored resources. But in some cases, the question remains, despite the use of the best resources. The patient can no longer bear their deteriorating health, the loss of independence and being completely bedridden or sick with no hope of improvement. Articulate verbal patients certainly have an advantage. However, an experienced doctor should be able to determine quickly enough whether the request could have been prevented or not by asking pertinent questions and playing the devil's advocate, such as asking whether the patient would still want euthanasia if the nausea and vomiting were to stop. This type of gentle probing requires experience but also basic empathy, subtlety and a willingness to talk about the issue. If the attendant doctor does not feel comfortable doing it, they should consult a colleague with more experience, such as a LEIF doctor or a palliative doctor who is open to euthanasia.

For the patient, it is also crucial to know what their attendant doctor's views on euthanasia and palliative care are. These questions should be asked as early as possible in the illness so there is time to change doctor if views differ.

When the doctor and friends and family realise that the patient is sticking to their decision, the attendant doctor, out of respect for the patient, should start the required procedures (written request, second opinion, third opinion if necessary) or refer the patient to a different doctor.

It is also important to ascertain the patient's wishes in relation to the euthanasia (the place, people present etc.) and to explain the different ways that it can be done: an injection into the vein or a lethal drink.

Aftercare

Although many go on about the attention to bereavement in cases of euthanasia, it actually doesn't have to be any different from any other death. In an 'ideally' performed euthanasia, the processing of thoughts and emotions mostly takes place beforehand. Afterwards, the relief of the bystanders is palpable, 'pleasantly' surprised that it 'was just that', that it happened so serenely and that the patient died so calmly. This is in contrast to the often gruesome 'spontaneous' deaths experienced by other patients who do not have the chance for a proper farewell because the dying patient appears too confused, to be in too much pain or to be too dazed. This is not a plea for patients to choose to die by euthanasia, but an attempt to waylay the countless prejudices and misconceptions about it.

The doctor should also reassure family and friends that they are available the following week, month or even year to discuss the matter. In the vast majority of cases, this is not required, which further illustrates that euthanasia should be considered 'good medical practice'.

13　Difficulties in life-termination procedures

S ir Thomas More was an English humanist, jurist and statesman as well as a Catholic martyr who was beheaded in 1535. He was beatified in 1886 and canonised in 1935, 400 years after his execution. In his bestseller, *Utopia*, published in Latin in 1516, he wrote:

> As I told you, when people are ill, they're looked after most sympathetically and given everything in the way of medicine or special food that could possibly assist their recovery. In the case of permanent invalids, the nurses try to make them feel better by sitting and talking to them, and do all they can to relieve their symptoms. But if, besides being incurable, the disease also causes constant excruciating pain, some priests and governmental officials visit the person concerned, and say something like this: 'Let's face it; you'll never be able to live a normal life. You're just a nuisance to other people and a burden to yourself – in fact you're really leading a sort of posthumous existence. So why go on feeding germs? Since your life's a misery to you, why hesitate to die? You're imprisoned in a torture-chamber – why don't you break out and escape to a better world? Or say the word, and we'll arrange for your release. It's only common sense to cut your losses. It's also an act of piety to take the advice of a priest, because he speaks for God.' If the patient finds these arguments convincing, he either starves himself to death, or is given a soporific and put painlessly out of his misery. But this is strictly voluntary, and, if he prefers to stay alive, everyone will go on treating him as kindly as ever. Officially sanctioned euthanasia is regarded as an honourable death.

The above is in fact a plea, before its time, for palliative care, assisted suicide and euthanasia.

What is the difference between a terminal and a non-terminal patient?

If a patient is not expected to die in the foreseeable future, i.e. is non-terminal, a second and third (LEIF) doctor must be consulted (see p. 163) before euthanasia can be approved. In addition, a waiting period of one month between the signing of the written request and the euthanasia must be respected. And yet the difference between terminal and non-terminal is not very well understood. In certain extreme cases, it is very clear. An emaciated, bedridden and totally metastatic cancer patient weighing 40 kg can be considered terminal without hesitation. The same goes for a completely paralysed patient (as a result of a traffic accident) who requires artificial respiration and feeding, or an incurable psychiatric patient with severe mental suffering: both of them can be considered non-terminal. But between these two extremes are many patients whose life expectancy cannot be determined with any certainty. At what point does a patient become terminal? When they have only a few days to live? Or weeks? Or even six months, as specified in Lord Falconer's 'Assisted Dying Bill' in the UK? The best definition of the concept of 'terminal' is a definition given *a posteriori*: once someone has died, it is fair to assume that they were terminal beforehand. According to Belgian legislation, these decisions have wisely been left to the attendant doctor. In the Netherlands the law fortunately makes no distinction between terminal and non-terminal patients.

For patients who have requested euthanasia, this distinction can be a real problem. Quite a few healthcare facilities and doctors claim that they are prepared to perform euthanasia, but only on terminal patients. In so doing they are in fact adopting the position of the Christian Democrats (see box, p. 149). And therein lies the problem. It means that a doctor can refuse a request for euthanasia because the patient is not yet 'terminal'. The following example is certainly not an isolated case. A pulmonologist refers a patient with lung cancer, metastases in the brain, the liver and the skeletal system to another hospital. The patient makes repeated requests to be euthanised but the doctor decides that they are non-terminal and so the euthanasia cannot be performed in the hospital where the request was made. The doctor and the healthcare institution have the power on their side, are 'always right' and many patients are therefore in danger of having their requests rejected – hence the importance of the emergency consultation UL team (see below).

There is no obligation to refer cases

The pulmonologist in the example above who rejected the euthanasia request acted correctly when referring the patient to another institution. According to the Belgian Euthanasia Law, however, doctors are not required to refer their patients. They are merely required to inform patients in good time that they are not willing to honour their requests. It is up to the patient to find another willing doctor. This is not easy for a single, very weak, bedridden patient. The medical code of ethics requires continuity of care, but practice has shown that too many requests for euthanasia are ignored or unilaterally sidelined by an increase in painkillers and/or sedatives.

It was with these 'unheard' patients and for doctors wanting a second opinion that I – along with academics from the VUB, the University of Ghent, the University of Antwerp and the Catholic University of Leuven – founded a consultation team, UL team, in Wemmel in December 2011 to answer their end-of-life questions.* The team is also supported by the VUB's Dignified Life's End Chair.

Palliative sedation as an alternative to euthanasia

Palliative sedation has been mentioned several times, but is covered in more detail here because in practice it is often proposed as a 'better alternative' to euthanasia.

Palliative sedation entails inducing a dying patient with unbearable, untreatable complaints into an artificial coma so that they no longer consciously have to endure any suffering. This happens primarily in cases of severe shortness of breath, pain, nausea and vomiting, anxiety and delirium.

---

* See www.ulteam.be, with a section in French and in English; tel. +32 78 05 01 55.

Unlike euthanasia, however, the aim is not to shorten life but rather to keep the patient unconscious until they die 'spontaneously' from their illness.

Another important difference with euthanasia is that although palliative sedation should be induced with the patient's consent (for patients who are still able to be consulted), it can also be induced without their consent if the patient is no longer competent to give consent. Consider a patient with a terminal brain tumour who is permanently confused, in pain and continually vomiting. A doctor in this instance will clearly assume responsibility and give the patient sufficient pain medication and sedatives to stop the suffering despite the fact that consultation with the patient is no longer possible. As a result, doctors are comfortable administering palliative sedation and they would rather sedate patients (even those who are fully competent) without consultation than reply to a request for euthanasia: the (legal) procedure is much simpler.

Palliative sedation is therefore still too often proposed as an alternative to euthanasia, even in countries with euthanasia laws. A patient may ask for euthanasia, but the doctor will talk them out of it with comments such as 'It's still too early for euthanasia' and recommend palliative sedation instead. The weak, debilitated patient is forced to agree with this recommendation – which is a violation of both their human and patient rights.

It frequently happens that after days of palliative sedation, when the visiting family is exhausted and wanting it to end, the doctor changes their intention and progressively increases the doses of hypnotics to help 'nature take its course'. In fact, the doctor in this instance has just performed 'life termination without request' (see p. 139), but to the outside world it is still referred to as 'palliative sedation'.

It has already been noted that the number of palliative sedations has almost doubled (8–15 per cent of all deaths) since the introduction of the Euthanasia Law in 2002. This is probably due to greater focus on and empathy for terminal suffering. But these figures also undoubtedly cover unanswered requests for euthanasia. Perhaps this is also the case in the UK, where the number of palliative sedations is estimated to be even higher, i.e. 18 per cent of all deaths. It is also disturbing to note that the number of palliative sedations in French-speaking Belgium is twice as high as in Flanders. This may be due to French-speaking doctors adopting a more paternalistic attitude (conversely, 80 per cent of registered euthanasia requests come from Flanders).

Although theoretically the intention with palliative sedation is not to shorten the patient's life, in practice it is an inevitable side-effect. Either the patient is administered an under-dose and wakes up again, or they are given an overdose and die earlier than foreseen. The exact dose of sedative drugs to keep the patient continuously sedated without shortening their life is impossible to determine without continual monitoring of their vital functions (which only happens in anaesthetics, during surgery for example).

Given the above observations, it is only logical, out of respect for human and patients' rights, that registration of palliative sedation be made obligatory in the same way as euthanasia. It is noteworthy that opponents of the Euthanasia Law have not reached this conclusion themselves; neither do they support the idea.

At the end of 2013 the Medical Board of the University Hospital Brussels unanimously approved the motion to register all palliative sedations performed in the hospital to create transparency and to promote awareness among doctors.

The limitations of the anticipated declaration of intent

Many Belgians are extremely disappointed to learn that the current legal protection against future suffering is very limited. A patient in an irreversible coma can only request euthanasia by means of an anticipated 'declaration of intent'. No provisions are made for *affected* brain functions such as persistent confusion from brain metastases, seriously damaged brain activity following a massive brain haemorrhage or Alzheimer's (dementia). These irreversible brain damages seem to attract much interest. It is also noteworthy that the Law on Patients' Rights establishes that patients can specify beforehand that in the event of the above-mentioned brain damage, any life-prolonging treatment – including the administration of food and fluid – must be stopped. Someone with an extensive cerebral infarction can be allowed to starve to death – if the patient has previously specified it in writing – but in the same circumstances one is not allowed to act on a previously written request for euthanasia.

It becomes even more Kafkaesque when a patient suddenly – i.e. not by means of an anticipated declaration of intent – is allowed to request euthanasia at the *onset* of dementia: the patient is still fully capable of discernment but suffering unbearably from the realisation that in a few months this will no longer be the case. The famous Flemish writer and poet Hugo Claus, who was nominated for the Nobel Prize in Literature, took advantage of this opportunity in the spring of 2008 and made it public. The 'Claus effect' certainly made an enormous impact.

Echoing earlier legislative proposals by, among others, senators Jeannine Leduc, Paul Wille (Liberals), Myriam Vanlerberge and Christel Geerts (Socialists), new proposals were put forward in 2008 by Jean-Jacques De Gucht and Paul Wille which also dealt with other loopholes, such as the limited validity of the euthanasia declaration of intent (maximum five years), euthanasia for minors capable of discernment and life termination of newborn babies (see also the Groningen Protocol, p. 194).

As already mentioned, the proposal to extend the Belgian Euthanasia Law to minors capable of discernment – provided certain conditions are met – was voted into law by a large majority in February 2014.

The difference between a written request, a positive declaration of intent and a negative declaration of intent

Many people confuse these three definitions:
- A written request is, in fact, putting into writing a current request for euthanasia. It may be written on any piece of paper, even on the same day as the euthanasia is performed (on a terminally ill patient).
- A positive declaration of intent is a term used in the Euthanasia Law. An example can be downloaded from www.health.fgov. be/euthanasie or can be found in the LEIF brochure (see p. 161). People can use it to express an *advance* desire to be euthanised in the event that they should fall into an irreversible coma. It is valid for a maximum of five years and therefore needs to be updated regularly.

Since 1 September 2008, this (euthanasia) declaration of intent can be registered with the local authorities.

- A negative declaration of intent (formerly referred to as a 'living will') does not fall under the Euthanasia Law but under the Law on Patients' Rights. Patients can use this form to express an *advance* desire to refuse certain treatment should they later be unable to express it, hence the name 'negative' declaration of intent. It frequently concerns discontinuing treatments such as the artificial administration of food and liquids. An example of a negative declaration of intent can be found in the LEIF brochure (see p. 161).

'Anything not covered by the Euthanasia Law is potentially murder'

It has already been demonstrated several times that 'good medical practice' such as pain relief or mercy killing is often confused with euthanasia, or worse, with murder. The prosecutions of doctors in Boom, Ronse and Ostend and also the accusation against Dr Bonnemaison in Pau in France at the beginning of 2014 prove this all too well. When certain medical procedures are unclear there are better ways to clarify them than to drag the doctor in question through the law courts. Of course, not all end-of-life decisions can be regulated by law. Each case is unique and different and, moreover, it might not work in practice. A possible solution would be to make it compulsory to register all end-of-life treatment (particularly palliative sedation) in the same way as euthanasia. In anticipation of such a move, I have already mentioned that the Medical Board of the University Hospital Brussels at the end of 2013 specified that all palliative sedations be registered. This information is scientifically processed by Vicky Van de Velde, a member of the support team.

These problems could also be solved by universal use of codes of conduct such as DNR ('do not resuscitate') codes, which should preferably be discussed and agreed with the patient. It is possible to do this while working through the advance care planning (ACP) programme in the

LEIF brochure, which contains all the necessary, ready-to-use legal forms (see p. 161).

Meanwhile, the good practice of pain management and palliative care are again being compromised by all these prosecutions and intimidation.

In conclusion, would it be better to set up a commission, similar to the Belgian Federal Euthanasia Committee, to decide on all disputed end-of-life decisions and also to examine all registered decisions, such as palliative sedation? Complaints relating to the stopping of treatment, for example, could then be referred to this commission, which would assess the case before the public prosecutor is notified, and the doctor is accused of murder, with all the negative consequences.

14 Bereavement and bereavement care

Bereavement is an essential emotional response to loss. It is the debt that must be paid before being able to enjoy life again. In this chapter I will focus primarily on the elements of the grieving process after someone we care for dies after a long illness.

Mourning is normal. And yet its inclusion in the new *Diagnostic and Statistical Manual of Mental Disorders* (*DSM-5*) has resulted in a lot of protest. Although there are characteristics common to all grieving, reactions differ greatly from individual to individual. The length of the grieving process, the various stages, their order and the way in which people mourn are indeed very personal. These differences depend on the way in which the loved one died (whether or not you were able to bid farewell), the nature of the relationship, any additional stress such as changing job, caring for small children etc.

And, of course, we must not forget that there are people who do not express their emotions, who do not mourn. This type of reaction does not necessarily cause any problems.

Healthcare professionals must, above all, be able to prevent 'normal' mourning from developing into a complicated grief process. They must also be able to recognise early warning signs that a person's grief is spiralling out of control in time to refer the bereaved to a grief therapist.

Unfortunately, 'grief therapist' is not a protected title and there are many charlatans out there who, having been trained for a few weekends, feel qualified to put a sign on their door reading 'grief therapist' or 'mourning specialist'.

Inadequate care of complicated grief can have disastrous consequences (in a similar way to dubious alternative medicine). A person who has not followed sound basic training such as a psychology degree with additional specialisation in bereavement therapy should not be allowed to hold the title 'therapist'.

Healthcare professionals should be able to recognise 'normal reactions' to loss in order to support the bereaved and diagnose a complicated grieving process in time.

Common reactions to loss:

- Behaviour:
    - disorganisation;
    - lethargy or apathy;
    - cherishing of objects belonging to the deceased;
    - dreaming about the deceased;
    - looking for the deceased;
    - visiting places that evoke memories of the deceased;
    - avoiding remembering the deceased;
    - sighing;
    - loss of appetite;
    - crying;
    - restlessness;
    - disturbed sleep;
    - antisocial behaviour;
    - absent-minded behaviour.
- Feelings:
    - relief;
    - periodic suicidal feelings;
    - loss of hope, faith, reason to live;
    - feeling 'broken' or 'dislocated';
    - feeling that the world is unreasonable, unpredictable and dangerous;
    - crisis of faith;
    - isolation, feeling lost;
    - despair, yearning for the deceased;

- loneliness, hopelessness;
- violent mood swings, irritability;
- anxiety and depression;
- feelings of guilt and self-blame;
- anger with the deceased for dying, with the doctor who 'caused' the death, with God for allowing it;
- shock and numbness;
- sadness.
- Cognitions:
  - disbelief;
  - denial of the death;
  - short aural and visual hallucinations (for example hearing the deceased's voice);
  - feeling the deceased's presence;
  - confusion and difficulty concentrating.
- Physical sensations:
  - feeling of depersonalisation;
  - loss of energy;
  - muscle weakness;
  - shortness of breath;
  - headache, abdominal pain and nausea;
  - dry mouth;
  - oversensitivity to noise;
  - 'empty' stomach;
  - tight chest and throat.

All these reactions are possible, although the order may vary. It is also possible to experience them before the loss of a loved one, for example after learning of the terminal diagnosis. This is known as 'anticipatory mourning'.

These reactions are considered normal unless they lead to total disarray or remain *unchanged* over a period of months or years.

A normal mourning process (*with reactions that change and evolve*) can, nevertheless, last for many years after the loss.

Healthcare professionals, with their knowledge and understanding of these symptoms, are able to reassure mourners by 'normalising' their reactions. By listening to them and confirming that these reactions are normal, mourners can be guided through the four classic mourning tasks, as identified by the American psychologist and grief therapist J. William Worden. These are:

- accept that the loved one really is dead;
- work through (process) the pain of the loss;
- adjust to a world without the deceased, find a reason to live without the deceased;
- find an enduring connection with the deceased while continuing to live.

Of course the healthcare professional can neither force the bereaved to undertake any of these tasks nor exert any time pressure on the bereaved.

It is important, however, to remain alert for any possible derailment in complicated reactions. Certain factors may make a person more susceptible to complicated mourning, including:

- The way in which the deceased died: suddenly without saying goodbye or physically wasted, surrounded by drips and probes due to therapeutic obstinacy. For some people, the ritual of saying goodbye is very important, whether it is a simple squeeze of the hand or performing the last rites.
- The nature of the deceased: a child, for example.
- The nature of the relationship with the deceased: if the deceased was a source of the bereaved's self-esteem or sense of worth or if the bereaved had been heavily invested in the role of full-time carer for the deceased during their illness.
- The bereaved's past history: how were previous experiences of loss dealt with, the presence of a mental disorder such as depression, more than one death in short succession, as happens in the case of AIDS in certain homosexual environments.
- The bereaved's personality: alcohol or drug abuse, anxiousness, low self-esteem and general distrust.
- Social factors: frequent moves leading to a limited social network or estrangement from the family.
- Triggering stress factors: unemployment, divorce etc.

The presence of these factors fortunately does not automatically imply that the person will experience a complicated grieving process.

Complicated grief and the corresponding symptoms manifest themselves primarily as:

- chronic bereavement, such as anger or depression which lasts for months or years without any change;
- delayed grief: suppressed feelings of grief which years later can provoke disproportionate reactions to minor incidents or an inability to speak about the deceased without excessive sadness;
- masked grief, in which the bereaved does not recognise the symptoms: unexplained anxiety or depression, panic attacks, chronic changes in lifestyle, avoidance behaviour, for example refusing to go to funerals or cemeteries;
- self-destruction: drugs and alcohol;
- exaggerated mourning: the bereaved recognises the symptoms but is unable to control them: anxiety attacks, difficulty concentrating, despair, feelings of worthlessness, phobias, manic behaviour and suicidal behaviour.

Fortunately, complicated grief is not common. Healthcare professionals should be careful to avoid trigger factors such as therapeutic obstinacy or not allowing for a proper farewell. Empathic listening, whereby normal grief reactions can be expressed is essential, where the loss is discussed and the suffering caused by the grief is validated. In addition, it is important for the bereaved to feel they have a safe environment where asking for help is not perceived as shameful.

Studies show that mourning after euthanasia is no different from the mourning process after death from other causes. In addition, with euthanasia the time of death can be planned so that the goodbyes from friends and family can be as comfortable and positive as possible. The Belgian Euthanasia Law respects patients' rights, in that only family members designated by the patient may be informed in advance of the euthanasia. Nevertheless, it is desirable that the most key family members be informed. It is important that the patient has good reasons for not doing so.

15 Senseless medical treatment: the problem of therapeutic obstinacy

You do not fail if you fail to cure;
You only fail if you fail to care.

During the hearings in the Senate following the introduction of the Euthanasia Law of 2002, people's views of suffering, palliative care, end-of-life decisions and death changed in an imperceptible way. The introduction of the law contributed to the demystification of death and the taboos surrounding it. The current end-of-life debate is the logical culmination of half a century of experience with cutting-edge medical equipment which can prevent a lot of human suffering, but also, if sustained for too long, can cause additional suffering.

Medical developments certainly attract a lot of attention.

The importance of this will be put into context below, as will the influence exerted by the qualified user of this technology (the doctor as the 'exorcist' of death) on global public health. Later, I will look into the arguments as to why so much futile treatment is still taking place.

The evolution of medical technology

The body, not the doctor, heals the sick. (Hippocrates)

Before the discovery of Aspirin® in 1899, the most important drug was the doctor. They were a kind of magician who, apart from questionable bloodletting and substandard use of morphine extracts, had nothing to offer in the way of therapy, except to add a magical element to the nursing of the sick. Or, put another way, the doctor played the role of a placebo, which was enough for the profession to acquire an important social status. Doctors had the exclusive right to issue death certificates, without which a person was not considered officially dead.

Towards the end of the nineteenth century the first germs, such as the Koch bacteria, were discovered thanks to the development of the microscope. However, this was only a diagnostic triumph, independent of any therapeutic possibilities.

The first antibiotics and anaesthetics were discovered around 1930, marking the advent of modern therapeutic medicine. Between 1930 and 1960 more than four thousand medicines were registered, although according to the US Food and Drug Administration (FDA), only 40 per cent of them were effective.

From the 1950s, new technical possibilities were established, particularly in the field of surgery. Between 1960 and 1980 there were a number of transitions: biochemistry to 'genetic counselling', the acceptance of Albert Einstein's theory of relativity and the transition into the computer age.

And finally in the 1980s came so-called groundbreaking medical techniques. The era of high tech saw the introduction of CT scans, in-vitro fertilisation, organ transplants, recombinant DNA technology and tube feeding. It is clear that in the West this was a key factor in the main focus of health being moved from home to the hospital. It would hardly be practical for family doctors to install PET scanners in their back gardens.

Throughout this evolution, questions were undoubtedly asked about the impact that these discoveries would have on the *general* public's health. The question now is whether the explosion of medical technology has had a positive influence on public health.

Below are some examples to illustrate these concerns. The intention in doing this is for the sake of critical analysis and certainly not to negate past efforts.

What about the discovery of medicines?

In 1812, the death rate in Europe from tuberculosis was at its peak: seven fatalities per 100 inhabitants. By the time Robert Koch discovered the tubercle bacillus in 1882 (subsequently named after him) the number of deaths was already in decline and had reached its lowest point by the time the first sanatoriums were established in 1910. The mortality rate decreased even further before the use of antibiotics against TB.

On the other hand, we know that as a result of the overuse of antibiotics over many years, many multidrug-resistant bacteria now exist which are responsible for at least half of all hospital-acquired infections in the USA, at a cost of more than $5 billion to society each year.

A similar story can be told about the development of chemotherapeutic agents against cancer. A very important discovery was made just after the First World War when it became clear that the poisonous 'mustard gas' which had been used as a weapon during the war prevented human cells from dividing. This product was later renamed 'mustine' and can be considered an ancestor of many chemotherapy drugs. There are currently some eighty products on the market, many of which were developed before 1970. And yet despite all these therapeutic efforts, the cancer mortality rate increased by more than 5 per cent a year between the early 1970s and the early 1990s.

Is there a general explanation for these observations? According to epidemiologists, the best way to reduce the spread of infectious diseases and epidemics is by introducing better hygiene, such as sanitary facilities and nutrition. This applies to the spread of TB, which has now reduced dramatically as a result of improved living conditions and not from taking medicines. The fact that TB is again prevalent, particularly among the North African population, despite the availability of tuberculostatic products, is largely due to the poorer hygienic conditions in which these people have to live.

The main cause of the rise in cancer mortality is due to excessive tobacco use, poor diet and widespread pollution.

What about the discovery and use of new medical techniques?

One would be justified in asking how new medical techniques can promote general public health. In-vitro fertilisation will not increase the birth rate of the general population, heart transplants do not reduce the incidence of heart disease and the machinery in the intensive care unit does not increase the average maximum age of the Western population.

There are those who claim that the bordering-on-hysterical widespread screening for prostate cancer in the USA is counterproductive. It creates a very real danger that many futile operations will be performed, as many men get prostate cancer at an advanced age without any risk to their health. Early detection of these occult cancers often leads to pointless but major surgery which can result in impotence and incontinence.

Some of the observations mentioned above have, for some people, led to a so-called anti-intellectualism and an aversion to scientific and technological development. This view is supported by other data, examples of which will follow.

The danger of anti-intellectualism

Bangladesh has more than a hundred and fifty million inhabitants but only one old source of cobalt used for irradiating cancer, a disease that affects at least one in four people there. In addition, the radioactive source for this device has not been replaced since 1965. This leads some people to question the usefulness of developing innovative technology when it is not available for most of the world's population.

One of the few real breakthroughs in chemotherapy is in paediatric oncology. In this domain 50 per cent of cancer patients are cured definitively following treatment. But here again, questions are asked about its relevance when it is known that over 80 per cent of all children live in the developing world and are not eligible for this type of treatment.

Such anti-intellectual tendencies should be avoided. Without further scientific research, we will be reduced to ignorant compassion (such as that of Mother Theresa in Calcutta) or even worse, acting in ignorance without empathy. By this I mean that taking care and possibly curing the sick, anywhere in the world, is more than just holding hands out of pity. All initiatives in this domain must be based on scientific data. Public health is greatly improved through collective scientific knowledge, and epidemics can be prevented by the provision of uncontaminated drinking water and vaccination programmes.

The *overall* standard of health in a society depends very much on simple measures that have been introduced thanks to scientific knowledge, such as pure drinking water, uncontaminated meat, and sanitary facilities connected to sewage systems. This standard is not much affected by *individual* consumption of cutting-edge medical technology. The impact of attendant doctors and other expert users of this advanced technology on the *general* standard of health is therefore limited.

On the other hand, it cannot be denied that a CT scan – although expensive – has definitely not dehumanised the life of the individual patient. It saves countless people from painful and difficult examinations. Intensive care can often be life-saving for certain people and in-vitro fertilisation has improved the quality of life of infertile couples. In our industrialised society, the availability of medical technology therefore contributes to *individual* living standards, while the *general* standard of health in a society depends on collective measures such as better sanitation, healthier diets and the fight against pollution.

'Faith' in medicine is and will continue to be based on individual successes. Faith in medical technology can be seen as a modern form of religion. The first heart transplant, performed by Dr Christian Barnard, was perceived by the world, even in the slums of Calcutta, as a victory for man over nature. The operation received the same overwhelmingly enthusiastic response as the first landing on the moon. People know (consciously or subconsciously) that a heart transplant or a moon landing is something that not everyone will experience, but it illustrates how deeply ingrained our belief in today's technology is.

A pill for every ailment

As previously mentioned, doctors have to focus on individual successes. They are still trained to apply high technology expertly and autonomously, often with little concern for the patients' real needs.

Doctors have thus evolved from being powerless placebos to the providers of high-tech amenities. Doctors now find a remedy for every illness, for fear of being perceived as inadequate. Even issues that would be better addressed on the social level are medicalised individually by doctors and reduced to lengthy drug treatments, as illustrated by endless consumption of statins and antidepressants. The WHO predicts that depression will be the disease of the twenty-first century, a fact that is skilfully used by the medical industry. By *marketing fear*, simple threats are promoted to diseases.

Experience shows that patients at the end of their lives often continue to be treated until the therapeutic arsenal is fully 'exhausted'. In the 'best' case this is then followed by comfort (palliative) care or a decision is taken concerning the end of the patient's life. Patients are often treated for too long and the alternatives are proposed far too late, at which point the patient is 'dumped' – excuse the expression – on palliative teams. It is ridiculous that treatment should be continued until death. This cannot be construed as treatment, but rather *abuse* or *therapeutic obstinacy*. Consider, for example, patients for whom doctors are considering which type of chemotherapy to use on one day and deciding to give them a drip with an overdose of painkillers and sedatives the next. In both cases, this is often done without consulting the patient.

As the disease progresses, depending on its evolution and taking into account the patient's wishes, doctors should gradually reduce active treatment, including the administration of food and liquids, to make way for more supportive treatment. This is to avoid having to interrupt active treatment abruptly to replace it with palliative care. The two options are not mutually exclusive. Patients who are receiving active treatment are also entitled to professional supportive care.

What is therapeutic obstinacy?

Therapeutic obstinacy should, in theory, be easy to define. It is the persistent administration of medical treatment even when it no longer serves any purpose, and can even be harmful to the patient. In practice, however, it is not always easy to know *in advance* whether a particular treatment *with hindsight* would have served no purpose. Some professionals claim to recognise therapeutic obstinacy when confronted with it but they are unable to define any general rules that can be applied.

Medical ethics

Medical ethics have been dominated for two and a half thousand years by the Hippocratic oath. However, this oath has been made completely obsolete by the advent of cutting-edge medical technology and modern thinking, and now the oath has only folkloric value. For example, according to the oath, doctors are required to make promises to multiple gods such as Apollo, Asclepius and Hygieia: not only to protect life at all times and not to abort unborn children but also not to perform any surgical interventions or to have sex with the patient, 'not even slaves'.

The extensive changes on social, political, economic, legal and medical levels that took place after 1900 led to the adoption of new views about ethical decision-making. It was also realised that the medical profession and the clergy were not the only people who could determine biomedical ethical principles, and that the dynamics of a changing society also needed to be taken into account. As medical technology advances, we are increasingly confronted with new issues. In the 1980s, biomedical ethicists, philosophers and church leaders reached a consensus on four major ethical principles.

Principle 1: beneficence – act in a way that benefits the patient

This principle is synonymous with Hippocrates's obligation always to act in the interests of the patient, and as such would definitely advocate good pain and symptom control as well as psychosocial and spiritual support.

With the advent of cutting-edge medical technology such as ventilators and artificial feeding machines, the question also arose of when and how long these treatments should be continued for the good of the patient. It should be noted that technical aids are ethically neutral and offer neither suffering nor relief. Only by carrying out a particular medical intervention on a given patient will it be possible to determine whether it contributes to their welfare. This requires good communication between patient and doctor: the patient can only decide on a given treatment after being informed of all the pros and cons. The doctor may only choose a particular treatment once the patient has approved it, unless of course no communication is possible. The doctor–patient relationship takes precedence over the doctor–machine relationship.

Principle 2: non-maleficence – do not harm, 'Primum non nocere'

This principle is also synonymous with Hippocrates's obligation to do no harm. It's a warning not to abuse medical power and knowledge. Doctors must not work sloppily nor cause any suffering disproportional to the problem. They should *not* insist that every patient must always be confronted with their imminent death, nor remove all hope or sedate patients unnecessarily.

Principle 3: autonomy – respect for the right to self-determination

When making decisions that have an impact on patients' welfare and interests, it is important to recognise their freedom and respect their choices. This means that patients must be informed: choices can only be made when all the options are known. Choosing not to choose is also a choice. As long as the patient can be consulted, doctors must not make unilateral decisions. Patients also have the right to refuse treatment, as was confirmed in the 2002 Patients' Rights Act. This does not mean that patients are entitled to claim disproportionately expensive or futile treatments. This goes against the 'do no harm' and 'justice' principles. One person's freedom stops where another person's freedom begins.

Principle 4: justice – the fair distribution of resources

This ethical value is a fairly recent development. It is based on the fact that the healthcare budget is not infinite and therefore available resources must be distributed fairly. This is necessary not only to protect weak patients but also to safeguard the welfare of society. The major challenge is to identify and stop futile treatment so that the freed resources can be usefully used for good end-of-life care (which is still underresourced) among other things. The conclusion of the first report by the Belgian Federal Palliative Care Evaluation Committee in May 2005 highlights this problem. If this reasoning is extrapolated worldwide then it is clear that there is still a lot of work to be done before this principle becomes universal.

These principles do not, however, guarantee that the correct decision will be made in daily practice. Neither do they provide any guidance when there is a conflict of ethical values. According to the principle of beneficence, a patient who is in agony should be given enough morphine to relieve the pain but if this will shorten the patient's life it comes into conflict with the second principle, 'do no harm'. Artificial ventilation is meant to promote wellbeing (principle 1). However, this can turn into a breach of principle 2 – no harm – if the ventilation is sustained for too long. The correct decision in each case depends on the patient's specific clinical, biographical and cultural data and the wisdom of the parties involved.

What is futile medical treatment? In acute, curable or reparable conditions, this question is only asked in cases of *overconsumption* of diagnostic or therapeutic medicines: for example, administering antibiotics, which are only effective on bacteria, for a viral infection is senseless. The correct medical response to an inguinal hernia is corrective surgical intervention, although it is also possible to apply the *wrong* treatment (not to be confused with *futile* treatment). A 'medical error' can lead to complications, but this has nothing to do with therapeutic obstinacy. The adverse consequences are caused by unforeseen circumstances or by inadequate professional knowledge.

The success rate of the different options for treating chronic or life-threatening conditions is rarely 100 per cent and depends on various factors.

Chronic pain caused by damaged vertebrae as a result of arthritis could possibly be treated by the orthopaedic fixation of several vertebral bodies. The orthopaedic surgeon should discuss the pros and cons with the patient.

The more life-threatening a condition is, the greater the chance that therapeutic obstinacy becomes real and the less the doctor tends to be willing to engage in dialogue. People tend to favour treatment, even with a very limited success rate: not treating a patient is worse because it results in death. As a result, treatment of patients is exaggerated because dying is not an option. Death is still too often considered a failure of medicine or a lack of professionalism. As a result, patients die lonely, attached to a machine or drip.

Therapeutic obstinacy is a result of the derailment of the interaction between patient, environment and doctor.

Patient

Doctors certainly do not deserve to take all the blame. Certain patients with life-threatening conditions insist on futile treatment because of:
- fear of the dying process or dying;
- fear of death itself, separation anxiety;
- an underlying psychological problem, for example an unresolved family conflict;
- insufficient information;
- mythical belief in high technology.

Environment

The patient's environment is not limited to family but also includes the hospital or residential care centre where the patient is being treated. The family may share the same views as the patient. The hospital or residential care centre may prolong treatment for economic reasons.

Doctor

Doctors persist with treatment for the following reasons:
- their conditioning as a result of their training/negative paternalism;
- unrealistic faith in treatment options;
- sense of duty, 'rescuers' syndrome;
- rationalisation of their own fear of death;
- fear of losing the patient's confidence/trust;
- lack of empathy;
- scientific or material interest;
- fear of prosecution for stopping treatment because of the confusion with euthanasia;
- insufficient or uncertain knowledge of the prognosis;
- insufficient knowledge of other possibilities such as palliative care;
- inadequate communication skills to get around a non-treatment decision.

To start with, doctors need to change their attitudes. One of the main problems is that is there is no nice way to tell a patient that their active treatment is no longer helping. Nevertheless, continuing treatment that has no physical advantage may still be psychologically important for the patient. Consultation is thus clearly necessary. The earlier this communication takes place and the more details provided by the doctor, the fewer problems there will be to resolve later.

Is there a remedy for therapeutic obstinacy?

The first step is to ensure that patients are given *accurate information*. In this, attendant doctors play a very important role, although information currently available via the internet and other media should not be underestimated. It undoubtedly empowers patients and their families. Of course, the media also provides a lot of misinformation. In addition, spectacular new treatment possibilities attract far more attention than regular daily care facilities and create unrealistic expectations that make calm consultations difficult and promote 'medical shopping'.

Advance guidelines are certainly important. And with an ageing population this advance care planning (ACP) will become more and more important. Patients have a right to complete information which will then allow them to specify, using a declaration of intent form, which treatment or examinations they no longer want in a particular situation. This information helps the doctor make a decision when communication is no longer possible, for example with dementia patients. According to the Belgian Patients' Rights Law, doctors are required to honour these refusals. These declarations of intent are best completed while the person is still healthy and not emotional as a result if being seriously ill. Unbiased objective information and the various legal documents are available in the LEIF brochure (see p. 161). Some residential care centres ask the future resident (and family) during registration about what treatment he/she would like in certain circumstances. This is a commendable initiative because it also prevents unnecessary hospitalisation. A declaration of intent requesting euthanasia has more restrictions and, in Belgium, can only be acted on when the patient has become irreversibly comatose.

Many hospitals have introduced the so-called DNR codes (do not resuscitate). They are meant as a written form of communication between healthcare professionals about what treatment they are restricted to if the patient is in a given state. This is a useful guide for the doctor on call to make an acceptable decision in an emergency situation. For example, use of these codes can prevent a patient with generalised cancer and brain metastases who falls into a coma from being unnecessarily resuscitated. Obviously the use of these codes is best discussed with the patient beforehand, although this unfortunately doesn't usually happen due to the hectic nature of a hospital. In addition, the codes often differ from hospital to hospital. Finally, a similar system should also be introduced in home care and nursing homes, to prevent unnecessary hospitalisation by the GP on call.

Promoting interdisciplinary dialogue can also reduce the number of futile treatments. It also helps form a better picture of the patient and their needs.

Changes to medical training are fundamental – not so much the content of the training but the way in which it is taught. Doctors should not be trained to look automatically for treatment or diagnostic resources but also to look for whether a patient who has reached a certain stage of a given condition requires treatment at all.

Finally, there must be a shift of resources in the social-security system. It currently focusses largely on funding for technical developments and their use, which by definition promotes over-consumption and over-treatment. There are, however, clear opportunities to combat therapeutic and diagnostic obstinacy: better remuneration of non-technical applications such as interdisciplinary dialogue, better remuneration of palliative care, support for initiatives that promote home care, such as palliative day-care units, introducing treatment guidelines, punishing the use of expensive alternatives when a cheaper option is available and close monitoring of over-consumption. However, the Government faces many powerful lobby groups which, for obvious reasons, advocate more and better refundable technology.

In 1998, a staff member of the Belgian national insurance system investigated the average cost of a patient's final hospitalisation, from the time of being admitted to the time of death. The average cost worked out to €15,000 per patient. When you consider that 60 per cent (sixty thousand) of Belgium's annual deaths take place in hospital, this adds up to an annual cost of €900 million. And yet 70 per cent of Belgians want to die at home. For every ten thousand patients who do not die in hospital, an additional €150 million is freed up for home-care support. This requires no further comment, particularly since most people would rather not be hospitalised.

Another example concerns the usefulness of setting up a Belgian Hadron-therapy Centre. This form of therapy is based on irradiation with charged particles such as protons, and may still offer relief to cancer patients who no longer qualify for classic radiation therapy. Pressure to build such a centre is particularly strong from French-speaking Belgium. The Belgian Health Care Knowledge Centre (KCE) was asked to examine the usefulness of such a centre in Belgium. The resulting report in 2007 claimed that just to build a Hadron-therapy Centre would cost in the region of €160 million. Given the high operating costs of such a centre, it would have to be able to irradiate 900 patients annually, which would add another €100 million to the annual running costs. First, it is estimated that a maximum of a hundred patients per year are prescribed Hadron therapy, and second, in many cancers it has not been shown to have any added value as it is usually used as palliative therapy. Finally, there are already several such centres in Europe (including one in the UK) which are happy to treat these hundred Belgian patients, and so one wonders whether it is worth pushing for such a centre to be built in Belgium.

The way to get better funding for palliative care is not by phasing out technical benefits, but rather by avoiding wasting resources on futile therapy, thereby automatically releasing more resources for alternative care. Either way, it is clear that the debate about support for palliative care is intrinsically linked to therapeutic obstinacy. Interestingly, a remarkable study by Jennifer Temel on this very subject was published in the prestigious *New England Journal of Medicine* in 2010. The study showed that the timely introduction of palliative care in lung cancer patients not only leads to less aggressive and expensive treatments, but above all to a better quality of life, and these patients even lived longer! So what are we waiting for?

Moreover, it complies with medical ethics principle 4: fair use of resources.

What about adult patients who are unable to express themselves?

Until now, I have spoken about personal autonomy and consultation with the patient. But what about patients who can no longer be consulted? Consider a dementia patient who screams from pain caused by pressure sores, or the countless elderly patients who struggle to communicate or who say that 'doctors know best and they should decide'. Just because a patient cannot be consulted there is no reason to deviate from the four basic principles of biomedical ethics. Their quality of life must be the priority and not professional self-development, for example.

In all cases, every effort should be made to engage in dialogue in an understandable language. If necessary, this can be with the family. And lastly, in response to the above, 'a doctor should treat patients who are unable to express themselves as if they were their own family'.

The dramatic cases of Terri Schiavo and Eluana Englaro

The media circus surrounding the two vegetative patients Terri Schiavo and Eluana Englaro, who were in comas and artificially fed for years, is a good illustration of the ridiculous proportions that therapeutic obstinacy can assume (see p. 141).

Decisions on whether to continue artificially administering food and liquids are taken every day in hospitals and certainly in residential nursing homes. I will discuss this here in a bit more detail as an example of how people continue with treatment that no longer serves any purpose.

Artificial feeding is a major medical procedure whereby a probe is placed in the patient's stomach or the administration of food and liquids is done through a vein or via a subcutaneous lead. It is not assisted feeding, in which a cup is held to the patient's mouth or moisture or liquid food is poured into the patient's mouth using a spoon or syringe.

Stopping artificial feeding is psychologically difficult, both for healthcare professionals and for the family. 'You must eat properly, or you'll get sick' and 'If you don't eat, you will die' are well-known sayings that explain why this decision is so difficult. It also means that any decision to start with artificial feeding must be carefully thought through. Once a gastronomy probe has been inserted, it is psychologically much more difficult to remove it. 'Think before you act.'

According to the ethical principle of 'beneficence' the artificial administration of food and liquids should benefit the patient. There are a number of reasons in favour of artificial feeding:

- Anorexia and loss of strength: loss of appetite, progressive weakness and weight loss can be very stressful. There are several possible treatments for anorexia-cachexia syndrome. In some specific cases, artificial feeding could be considered, for example, when there is an obstruction in the oesophagus caused by a tumour, or in some stages of HIV.
- Hunger/thirst/dry mouth: hunger is rare in terminal patients. Nevertheless, correctable causes of eating complications such as nausea, oral yeast infection and constipation must be treated. Corticoids stimulate

the appetite and are better phased out. Patients usually complain, not of thirst but of a dry mouth, which can easily be treated locally.

- Delirium/terminal agitation: this is a common end-of-life problem. In some cases, it can be helped by reducing the number of sedatives, treating an infection or constipation or correcting hypercalcaemia or hyponatraemia. Morphine-6-glucuronide (a morphine metabolite), for example, can result in cerebral toxicity in patients with reduced kidney function, resulting in impaired excretion of this metabolite. In such instances, liquid can still be administered through the vein or subcutaneously (about a litre of water daily – hypodermoclysis) to activate the kidney function.

- Fear of death: as already mentioned, the psychological impact of fear of death on the decision not to start with artificial feeding cannot be underestimated. Here again it is very important to listen to the patient and their family, to support them and tactfully discuss the advantages and disadvantages of artificial feeding with them. Sometimes the stress is so severe and the patient so concerned by not being able to eat that these discussions achieve little. The best stress reduction can be caused by administering – even when futile – small amounts of food through an existing gastronomy tube or even a nasogastric tube or by hypodermoclysis.

Artificial feeding can be harmful to dying patients, which is contrary to principle 2. It can cause distension of the stomach, nausea and vomiting, diarrhoea, shortness of breath and even aspiration pneumonia. Intravenous feeding and liquid administration can cause fluid accumulation in the lungs. It can even increase the risk of infection and reduce survival.

Out of respect for the right to self-determination (principle 3), the patient should be involved in the decision-making process as early as possible. Once the illness has reached a stage whereby patients are no longer able to express themselves, the families should be heard in these discussions. Obviously the importance of the existence of a prior negative declaration of intent cannot be over-emphasised.

From the above it appears that there is no one formula that fits all. It is known that artificially administering food and liquids is, in many circumstances, futile and can even be physically harmful. Nevertheless, sometimes administering a little liquid can significantly reduce stress.

What about severely disabled or critically ill newborn babies and children?

The Groningen Protocol

Another significant problem is the attitude towards seriously ill newborn babies and children in Belgium who are incapable of requesting euthanasia. This does not mean their suffering is any less. This debate again attracted a lot of public attention in 2006 after the publication of a letter in the newspaper *De Standaard* by Inge Verhelst in which she described the harrowing agony of her newborn baby who had serious irrevocable brain damage, meaning that she could never lead even a minimum of what philosopher Leo Apostel described as a 'typical human life' (having a social and individual identity, being able to act, choose and make decisions). Despite this fact, the medical team unilaterally decided to 'save' this baby's life at any cost. How desperate Verhelst and her husband must have felt when, in addition to the upheaval of seeing their seriously ill, traumatised newborn baby, they were sent from one part of the hospital to another. And now they will live with the consequences of the decisions that were taken from above for the rest of their lives. Inge Verhelst pleaded in her letter for the mercy killing of her child. The countless reactions to the letter showed just how much Belgian society was moved by this.

A more recent drama concerns baby Ella-Louise, whose image, broadcast on Belgian national television on 4 May 2012, still sticks in peoples' memories. It might also have sparked the debate on dignified death for minors in the Senate. Ella-Louise suffered from a rare incurable metabolic disorder, Krabbe's disease, which attacks the nerves and the brain, and she was going to die in the forthcoming weeks or months. There were two possible ways to treat her: life termination in an emergency or palliative sedation while stopping feeding. The second option was chosen, and her mother, Linda Van Roy, was asked to care for her baby herself.

This was such a gruesome experience for Linda (Ella-Louise wasted away completely and grimaced with pain while being washed) that she decided to film her suffering and make it public in the hope that it would not be repeated. It would have been more humane to apply the Groningen Protocol (see below).

In 2005, the medical world was 'rocked' by doctors Pieter Sauer and Eduard Verhagen of the Department of Paediatrics at the University Hospital Groningen. They had just published the 'Groningen Protocol' in the *The New England Journal of Medicine*. This protocol allows for the lives of children and newborn babies, unable to express themselves, to be terminated under certain circumstances. These children, who are born with serious defects such as complete brain damage from bleeding, are going to die after a few weeks or months of agony, or will never lead a typical independent human life. Sauer and Verhagen were tired, as were many other paediatricians, of having to perform 'clandestine' life terminations in order to prevent therapeutic obstinacy. The main motive was to prevent medical technology from creating additional suffering, or maintaining suffering. This means of course that we, as a civilised society with *existing* suffering – such as children and adults with profound mental disabilities (caused by non-congenital brain lesions or acquired brain damage for example) – should treat these cases with great care, which is, if we're honest, not always the case.

The proposal by Sauer and Verhagen to regulate formally the termination of the lives of minors could not be achieved by amending the existing Dutch Euthanasia Law since it is not 'euthanasia' (life termination at the request of the patient).

As a result of the Groningen Protocol – compiled by paediatricians at the University Hospital Groningen along with the Attorney General and the Ministry of Justice – Dutch doctors report all life-ending treatment for minors (not only newborns) who are unable to express themselves, according to a defined procedure: submitting a report of all treatment and decisions to the municipal coroner (in Belgium, the local medical examiner) and thus to the prosecutor (in Belgium, the public prosecutor). Each case is assessed within four to six weeks to determine whether the doctor acted with due care. If the response is positive, the hospital is not visited, neither are the parents questioned. These guidelines were adopted throughout the Netherlands afterwards. At the beginning of 2007, a Review Committee that makes recommendations to the prosecutor was established. This committee is composed of a health lawyer, an ethicist and a paediatrician.

I, along with the paediatricians of the University Hospital Brussels, am currently looking into whether this protocol could also be applied in Belgium. The Review Committee could be the same one that deals with other disputed end-of-life decisions (see Chapter 12).

16 Towards a new care culture

If you spend your whole life waiting for the storm, you'll never enjoy the sunshine.

Morris West

The terminology of two important concepts in end-of-life care appear to be working counterproductively in terms of their further evolution. Both the terms 'euthanasia' and 'palliative care' often have negative connotations.

The word 'euthanasia' has bad historical and emotional connotations because it is frequently associated with the Nazis' so-called 'Euthanasieprogramm' during which those considered inferior by the Nazis were killed (this was, however, *not at their request*). In addition, it is often used by the media and opponents to indicate other end-of-life decisions. Nevertheless, the term is now established and there is no alternative that describes *self-determined* death as succinctly. Either way, the term 'euthanasia' certainly didn't make the debate in Belgium straightforward. A similar misunderstanding of the word can currently be witnessed in other countries, sparking emotional reactions that are completely unrelated to the question. Consider the outcry over the question of whether or not to stop artificially feeding coma patient Eluana Englaro, which was incorrectly referred to by many media sources as Italy's *euthanasia* debate.

A similar problem occurs with the term 'palliation' or 'palliative care'. Non-healthcare professionals often associate the concept exclusively with terminally ill people, those who are suffering and the dying. Even doctors and other healthcare providers make this connection, and as a result either call in the palliative teams too late or not at all. From the definition of palliative care it appears that the distinction between curative medicine, palliative medicine and palliative care is paper thin and often artificial. Nevertheless, the difference is structurally maintained because the Belgian Government pays for palliative care only in the last phase of life. It is only paid for for a limited time, for example a flat palliative rate for two months. Palliative home teams, on the other hand, get a fixed amount per patient, regardless of the duration of the care. This also applies to the underpaid hospital teams and the palliative functions in residential care centres. Their overall activity is funded on an annual basis.

The palliative sector has regular discussions with the Belgian Government about the definition of a 'palliative patient' with regard to subsidy conditions. As a result, palliative-care professionals often feel they have to justify caring for an incurable patient for the legally allowed and therefore reimbursable amount of time. In this sense, it resembles the polemic of the euthanasia debate in which doctors are unable to distinguish between a terminal and a non-terminal patient. In the Euthanasia Law, this decision is left to the attendant doctor.

Of course it is also possible to reverse the question and ask instead what the definition of a 'curable patient' is. Again, as with the extremely strict repayment terms for palliative patients, this definition could be linked to the reimbursement system.

Healthcare, for a minority of people, consists of acute, curable diseases, while for the vast majority it consists of non-curable, chronic conditions, a fact that is not likely to change soon, given the ageing population.

Examples of chronic diseases are diabetes mellitus, rheumatoid arthritis, arthrosis, emphysema, chronic bronchitis, cardiac decompensation, arteriosclerosis, chronic hepatitis, chronic kidney failure, Crohn's disease, osteoporosis, HIV infection, multiple sclerosis, Parkinson's, Alzheimer's and various cancers.

Chronic diseases cannot be cured. It therefore makes sense to treat the disease and its symptoms as well as possible. This is in fact 'palliation' or 'palliative *medicine*'. Palliative medicine makes use of the same therapeutic and diagnostic arsenal that was developed for curative medicine. Thanks to recombinant DNA technology, massive amounts of human insulin can be produced to treat diabetes. Diabetes cannot be cured but daily injections of insulin can control the symptoms and complications so well that the patient can still live a high quality of life without their condition having any impact on life expectancy. Without insulin, diabetes can be a life-threatening condition for some patients, and even with insulin some diabetes patients develop complications. The same reasoning can be applied to other non-curable conditions such as the HIV infection and some cancers.

It is therefore difficult and in fact pointless to limit the length of time that these patients can be given the status of 'palliative'. It is also clear that the current definition of a curable patient is not very helpful.

With chronic problems, curing the patient is by definition not possible. The opinion of the palliative teams should therefore be sought as early as possible in the disease process. It is also for this reason that the WHO decided to change its definition of palliative care. Whereas it used to refer to 'care for incurable patients', the scope was changed in 2002 to 'care for life-threatening conditions'. Consulting the palliative teams early contributes to better prevention of worsening and future complaints.

Palliative care includes supportive care

It remains a reality that many cancer patients are averse to the concept of 'palliative' because they equate it with 'terminal', a sad reality, as a result of which many patients wait too long – sometimes indefinitely – before considering the potential benefits of this type of treatment. The above logic demonstrates that the adjective 'palliative' has many different layers, and for non-terminal patients could be better described as 'supportive'. It is unfortunate that some doctors maintain this aversion by dismissing patients who are considering these options with comments such as 'this type of care is not for you' or that it is 'far too early'. They are possibly trying to reassure their patients that they are not yet terminal, but in the meantime the damage is done.

The early introduction of the support (let's not even mention the word 'palliative') team allows the patient and family members time to become acquainted with the members of the team, and avoids the common 'palliative team = terminal team = death' association. It is clear from the above that there is no general rule to determine at what point these teams should be involved. It varies from patient to patient.

A new care culture in which 'palliative' is no longer synonymous with 'terminal'

Palliative care as a social movement needs to evolve more and more from 'terminal care' to a new care culture where illness is treated with empathy and in consultation with the patient at all stages of the disease (regardless of whether the patient still has a chance of being cured or has reached the palliative stage). This evolution calls for a seamless integration of the new care culture in the existing healthcare system, where the term 'palliative' is no longer synonymous with 'terminal' but also includes 'supportive'; support of incurable, not yet terminal, chronic diseases.

Patients and family will be placed back at the centre of the new care culture. This is not, however, as obvious as it seems. The phrase 'the patient is central' rolls too easily off the tongue and is generally considered just an expression.

The aim of healthcare based on the saying 'without sick people, there would be no need for healthcare providers' is indeed to provide the best environment for patients and their families. In practice, it is a bit different. The fact that patients are in very vulnerable positions due to their illness, be it physical (immobile) or psychological (unbearable anxiety), is not a reason for healthcare providers to abuse them. This would be all too easy. Their submissive, dependent position makes it very easy to impose things upon them, to ignore them, to patronise them, to keep them waiting, to prevent them from doing something. Seriously ill patients have enough to deal with with their illness, and they shouldn't be subjected to further frustrations in their mandatory relationship with healthcare providers. Instead, patients should be considered as full partners, admittedly with certain constraints. Adopting this attitude shows respect for the patient and can boost the corroded self-image. This is at least as important as all the so-called essential medical interventions.

Out of respect for the patient, it is important that they be engaged and consulted (or a family member if this is not possible) from the very first day of diagnosis. The quality of the very intense care during the terminal phase of life should also be applicable at all stages of the disease process, to a greater or lesser degree.

The Euthanasia Law has sparked a true (r)evolution in the doctor–patient relationship, and has had an incredibly emancipatory effect. Or perhaps it would be better to speak about a patient–doctor relationship, given that the patient is the main component in this relationship. Whereas in the past Belgian doctors were able to hide behind the illegal nature of euthanasia, now patients know that they have the *right* to ask for it. This is a real turnaround, because the increasingly empowered patient will want to see this right to decide about the end of their life extended to other areas of their healthcare. In addition, the recent Belgian Patients' Rights Law will provide patients with more support.

It should not be forgotten that consultation regarding end-of-life decisions is just the tip of the iceberg. Many decisions can be taken over the patient's head earlier in the illness, decisions that constitute human-rights violations.

17 Conclusion: how far have we come with end-of-life care?

Most people would rather die than think, in fact, they do so.

Bertrand Russell

We still have a long way to go. Barriers need to be broken down on a daily basis, undoubtedly because therapeutic obstinacy remains so dominant. Continually having to convince doctors may lead to mental fatigue. There is also a danger that palliative care teams prefer to work alongside regular care rather than to integrate themselves into it. The result is a bilateral hedgehog formation, resulting from the existence of two separate 'worlds': one in which healthcare professionals try and cure everything and the other where they think only about care. And as a consequence, there is frequently an absence of any consultation or cooperation, which obviously does not benefit the patient.

The challenges of the next decades

End-of-life care faces major challenges in the future. Firstly, there is an exponentially ageing population that will force us to develop new care facilities. The importance of good home care – supplemented by day centres – is therefore paramount. Not all older people will be able to go into residential care. This will also add to the importance of palliative care:

currently one in four people contract cancer; with the ageing population this is fast increasing to one in three. The same can be said of Alzheimer's Disease. This form of dementia increases with age, and it is estimated that from the age of 85, 30 to 50 per cent of people suffer from it. Training, especially for doctors, urgently needs to change: not so much the technical content but rather how to apply it.

If palliative care wants to be considered as an alternative to therapeutic obstinacy, then healthcare professionals must be able to engage in professional dialogue. This requires solid clinical knowledge based on scientific research. Science does not exclude empathy, but ignorance, albeit empathetic, will not help us to progress, and the level of care will remain that of Mother Theresa.

We are on the right track

Palliative care should not think that it is always right. Any self-criticism is probably not misplaced. Healthcare professionals who work intensively in palliative care may find themselves suffering from 'palliatitis'. This includes different 'symptoms', which is understandable, particularly for the generation who had to fight for the right of palliative care to exist. They may have a strong aversion to medical technology and possibly undertreat patients as a result. Their bedside manner may sometimes be too intrusive or patronising.

Also in the case of advance care planning, healthcare professionals should limit themselves to giving information and advice, and shouldn't want to dictate the path chosen by the patient. The LEIF brochure (see p. 161), out of respect for the patient's right to choose, has been prepared in this spirit: it provides objective information as far as possible, as well as all the necessary legal documents, ready for use without any sense of imposition. In this way (future) patients have the information to choose for themselves. And if they decide to leave the choice to the doctor because they will make the 'best' decision that is also a choice; deciding not to decide is a decision in itself.

Palliative staff often want patients to accept death and see it as a personal failure of their patient support if they are unable to achieve this. And yet, for the patient, to deny death is sometimes a way of dealing with a life-threatening condition in order to 'survive' mentally. This coping strategy is also common in healthy people: most of us live as if we are immortal and think about death as little as possible. There's nothing wrong with that as long as it does not cause any harm: an 85-year-old man should not be making twenty-year plans that have financial implications for himself and his descendants.

Palliative care providers often consider themselves to be part of a select palliative club as the only people to provide professional palliative care. The truth is that some of them are attracted to palliative care for strictly personal reasons, such as an incomplete bereavement process, and the process is more about helping themselves than the patient.

Hubris can be a dangerous pitfall. Palliative care cannot alleviate all misery. One shouldn't therefore try and resolve a thirty-year-old marriage problem in the last week of one's life, for example. Belief in the all-encompassing power of palliative care can even lead to 'palliative obstinacy'. In fact palliative care can follow the same mistaken logic that leads to therapeutic obstinacy. Therapeutic obstinacy is when doctors won't stop treatment even though the patient would benefit more from palliative care. We speak of palliative obstinacy when well-intentioned care is forced upon patients even though they don't want a 'deep meaningful' conversation or have in fact requested euthanasia.

It's all too easy to attribute the aversion that certain healthcare professionals have for palliative care to a denial of death and therapeutic obstinacy. In fact, it can also be due to palliatitis behaviour within the palliative sector.

Finally, palliative care needs to continue striving to improve the lives of seriously ill patients. As a social movement it must be careful not to make the same mistakes that many other reactive movements have made. Palliative organisations must not be seen as an end in themselves but as a means for seriously ill patients.

Another of the challenges facing us is to find a way to eliminate the polarisation that has grown up between the pro-palliative care and the pro-euthanasia camps.

Palliative caregivers frequently accuse the pro-euthanasia camp of portraying a frightening picture in which the benefits of palliative care are not mentioned. Conversely, euthanasia supporters tend to be suspicious of the (often religious) palliative care supporters who pretended before the Euthanasia Law came into force that, thanks to palliative care, they had never received any requests for euthanasia. The public debate at the time was about the way people wanted to die: without avoidable misery, possibly at a time of their choosing and preferably in their favourite place. Everyone agrees that the dying process should be dignified. Before the Euthanasia Law was introduced in Belgium, however, the concept of 'dignified' was interpreted differently by opponents of euthanasia.

Open-minded, receptive caregivers have long been aware that patients are not concerned with this. People who are suffering unbearably as a result of a medically hopeless situation just want to be helped. They are not interested in bombastic, ideologically tinted quotations. Neither are they interested in what healthcare professionals define as 'palliative care', 'end-of-life decisions' or 'euthanasia'. They just want a human solution to their specific problem.

Some fervent opponents of the Belgian Euthanasia Law, who, prior to the law's introduction used to claim that they were hardly ever asked about euthanasia, now admit that people are interested in the question. People now know that they have the *right* to talk about it, which is reassuring and can only improve end-of-life care. In fact it has come so far that these healthcare professionals now ask for additional funding because their workload has increased as a result of all the conversations about euthanasia. Nevertheless it seems that there are still those who continue to oppose the law and who seem to have little respect for different opinions or for the right to self-determination. This is apparent in the current acrimonious opposition to the extension of the Euthanasia Law – and in the emotional and rather conservative foreign press, where literally all possible means are used in an attempt to block any amendment of the law.

Euthanasia should not take precedence over palliative care, and vice versa. In Belgium, 80 per cent of euthanasia requests come from cancer patients and 80 per cent of patients cared for by palliative teams have cancer. In both instances we are talking about the same population. It shouldn't be so difficult in a pluralistic democratic society to convince dissident colleagues of the basic principle of palliative care, i.e. 'respect for people'. Healthcare professionals are entitled to their own personal beliefs – including about euthanasia – as long as they do not cause any harm to the patient. If this were to be the case, the patient should be referred to a colleague who holds different views.

Also, it is much more useful to invest this energy in combating therapeutic obstinacy. The conclusion of the first report by the Federal Evaluation Cell for Palliative Care in May 2005 is damning: 'one might well question an inclusive society where there are no restrictions imposed on the number of treatments a patient can be offered even though they achieve nothing and yet the budget for palliative care is severely restricted.' This conclusion is once again cited in the Federal Evaluation Cell for Palliative Care's report in May 2008, which means that there is still a lot to be done.

Everything can be reduced to the comment by my good friend and colleague Raymond Mathys, who in 2008, together with Jacqueline Herremans and myself, was awarded the Tenrei Ohta Laureate Award by the World Federation of Right to Die Societies: 'We should abandon the terms palliative care and end-of-life decisions (including euthanasia). They should all be replaced by one all-inclusive concept, namely 'a dignified life's end'.

Not only should the end of the dying process be dignified, but the whole process of the illness. The quality of dying in our society is still in stark contrast to our quality of life. Moreover, being sick should not mean waiting for death but rather getting the most out of life.

The pursuit of a dignified *life's end* includes both the pursuit of a dignified *life* and a dignified *end*.

Annex
Some tips on techniques and medicines

Treatment of early reactions after radiation therapy

Skin reactions

Eosin 2 per cent of an aqueous solution; Flammazine®.

Swallowing problems

Usually caused by an acute oesophageal infection after irradiation of the oesophagus, or possibly an opportunistic fungal infection: Nilstat® 4×1 drop per day.

Nausea and vomiting

Occurs when the stomach or intestines, or a large piece of the liver, are located in the field of radiation: metoclopramide (Primperan®) 4×10 mg per day.

Diarrhoea

Caused by irradiation of the bowel or rectum. Loperamide (Imodium®) after each loose bowel movement up to 8 times a day, or codeine. When patients are already being treated with morphine, then activated charcoal (Norit®) can be used.

Inflammation of mouth and throat mucosa

Oropharyngeal mucositis occurs after irradiation of the head-and-neck region. Acute problems can be treated with chlorhexidine (Hibitane®). Watch for a yeast infection (white spots). Mouthwash can also help.

Magistral mouthwash after irradiation
> Xylocaïne 400 mg
> Nystatine® 2.4 × 106E
> NaCMC 2 g
> Propylene glycol 15 ml
> Aqua ad 500 ml
> Mfsa 1 portion
> DT no 1 bottle
> S/ 6 × 1 tablespoon per day (rinsing and swallowing)

It is also possible to use iso-betadine and Nystatin (Nilstat® 4 × 1 drop per day). Bad breath is often caused by anaerobic bacteria. This can be treated with metronidazole, Flagyl® (3 × 500 mg per day), clindamycin or Dalacin C® (3 × 150 mg). Bleeding gums can be treated by rinsing the mouth with Exacyl® ampoules.

Pneumonitis

Can occur after irradiation of large surfaces of the lung. It is characterised by a dry cough and shortness of breath. The irradiation path can often be seen 'signed off' on the thorax x-ray. High doses of corticosteroids (Medrol® 1–2 × 32 mg) for 2–3 weeks, possibly combined with antibiotics to combat secondary infection.

Cystitis

Difficult to treat, but fortunately self-limiting. Possibly oxybutynin (Ditropan®) 4 × 5 mg per day against bladder spasms or medicine with an anticholinergic agent such as tricyclic antidepressants (Redomex®) or phenothiazines (Dominal®).

Pain treatment according to the WHO's pain ladder

Step 1: Weak non-opioids

For people with limited pain on the first step, non-morphine-like substances should be used. Prototypes are paracetamol (Dafalgan®), acetylsalicylic acid (Aspirin®) or any other NSAID (nonsteroidal anti-inflammatory drug), such as indomethacin (Indocid®), Ibuprofen®, Voltaren®, Apranax® and Celebrex®.

Paracetamol and acetylsalicylic acid are effective for about 4 hours. They should, in principle, be administered 6 times a day. NSAIDs last longer, and slow-release preparations also exist. In general they should be administered 2–3 times a day.

Acetylsalicylic acid (Aspirin®) reduces pain and fever at lower doses and may have an anti-inflammatory effect from just 3 g per day. It has a significant analgesic effect on bone metastases pain. The usual dose is 500–1000 mg 6 times a day, for example 1–2 500 mg Aspirin® pills 6 times per day. Many patients suffer from upset stomachs, especially at higher doses. This problem can be partially avoided by administering pills which are protected against stomach acid and whose content is released only in the small intestine, such as Acenterine®. Aspirin® effects blood clotting and should not be administered to patients with clotting problems. Very rarely the patient has a hypersensitivity reaction: allergic rhinitis, urticaria and bronchial asthma.

Paracetamol (Dafalgan®) similarly reduces fever but has no anti-inflammatory properties. The effective dose is between 500 and 1000 mg 6 times a day. It does not cause stomach upset.

Aspirin® is the prototype NSAID, but actually the category includes medications that have been developed since the discovery of phenylbutazone, i.e. indomethacin (Indocid®), Voltaren® and the more recent stomach-friendly NSAIDs that do not effect blood clotting, such as Celebrex® and Dynastat® (im-iv). NSAIDs like Aspirin® have an analgesic, anti-inflammatory and antipyretic effect and may even have a better effect than corticoids on cancer fever. Their anti-inflammatory effects mean that they are very effective on bone pain and inflammation around the tumour itself. Stomach upset is less pronounced than with Aspirin®. Patients who do not tolerate a particular NSAID should be prescribed a different one. Most NSAIDs cause constipation, but there are those which cause diarrhoea, such as Indocid® and Froben®. NSAIDs cause liquid and salt retention, thereby contributing to oedema formation and reducing the effect of diuretics.

When these products are administered correctly – the right dose at the right time – but the patient continues to feel pain then step 2 of the ladder, morphine preparations, is needed.

Since the products of step 1 work differently to morphine preparations, they could continue to be administered during steps 2 and 3.

Step 2: Weak opioids

The prototype is codeine. Alternatives are dihydrocodeine (Paracodin®), tilidine (Valtran®) and tramadol (Dolzam® and Dolzam®).

Codeine or methyl morphine is a weak morphine-like drug and is found in natural opium. It exhibits a similar working mechanism to morphine (which is 10 times more powerful) and is effective for a similar duration of 4 hours (with similar side-effects such as nausea, vomiting and constipation). Codeine can be combined with step 1 drugs such as acetaminophen. This is because morphine-like drugs work as analgesics in the central nervous system, in contrast to step 1 analgesics. Paracetamol and Codeine® is a known combined preparation with an effect that is more powerful than the sum of its parts. One to 2 pills can be administered 6 times a day.

Dihydrocodeine is up to twice as powerful as codeine. It is available in pill form (10 mg) and syrup (Paracodin®). Dosage: 5–20 mg up to 3 times a day.

Tilidine exists in drops and is very fast-working (after 10–20 minutes). Valoron® in addition to tilidine also contains the morphine antagonist naloxone to prevent misuse and addiction. When used in higher doses naloxone enters the general circulation and reduces the effect of tilidine. Valoron® serves no purpose and should not be used if the dosage needs to be increased, for example with terminal patients; neither should it be administered in conjunction with another morphine-like analgesic. Tilidine lasts 4 hours and is about 7 times less powerful than morphine and yet exhibits the same side-effects. One drop corresponds to 2.5 mg tilidine. It is pointless to administer more than 6×25 drops or 4×40 drops per day. It exists also in pill form and as a slow-release preparation effective for 12 hours.

Tramadol (Contramal®, Dolzam®) has a similar effect to morphine, but is 5 times less powerful and works for up to 8 hours. It has a different analgesic application point and would have a positive effect on neuropathic pain (see below). It is administered in 50–100 mg doses up to 6 times a day or as a long-acting preparation (12 hours). Tramadol is less constipating than morphine. It is available in the form of drops, capsules and suppositories.

If these analgesics do not effectively reduce pain it is necessary to move to the third and final step of the analgesic ladder: strong opioids, with or without step 1 analgesics. It makes no sense to administer step 2 weak opioids in conjunction with strong opioids. Codeine is therefore not administered at the same time as morphine because both have the same entry point.

There is also talk of a fourth step: the building of an epidural catheter with which to inject painkillers in or around the spinal fluid. In practice the indications for such an application are limited.

Step 3: Strong opioids

When other analgesics are no longer effective morphine must be administered. Unfortunately, there are many misconceptions and myths surrounding this substance.

Adjuvant substances or excipients

The so-called 'adjuvant' substances can be added on all steps (see p. 218).

How should morphine be administered?

1. Some important initial pointers

None of the recently discovered or synthesised opioids are superior to morphine. They all have similar side-effects. Their effectiveness usually lasts 4 hours or shorter. Some preparations are admittedly more powerful but with more side-effects. It is usually enough to increase the morphine dose to achieve the same effect. The only reason to use a different preparation is pronounced intolerance to morphine. Two interesting preparations are available on the market: hydromorphone (Palladone®) and oxycodone (Oxycontin®).

Finally, enduring myths need to be dispelled to allow for quicker and better use of morphine.

2. Oral morphine is preferable

When step 2 painkillers are no longer effective, morphine is administered orally. As with step 2, step 1 analgesics (for example NSAIDs) can still be used, with or without adjuvants.

Oral morphine can be taken in several ways: magistral syrup, drops or solution (Oramorph®) or in the form of slow-release pills such as MS Contin®. Morphine syrup works for 4 hours and must therefore be given 6 times a day. A higher dose of syrup (double dose) can be given before sleep to prevent the patient waking up from pain.

Morphine syrup is best prescribed in a concentration of 1 mg of morphine per millilitre of syrup. It prevents dosage errors: the number of millilitres of syrup consumed is equal to the number of milligrams of morphine ingested. A classic magistral prescription looks like this:

R/morphine hydrochloride 300 mg
orange blossom syrup 100 ml
aqua ad 300 ml
MFSA 300 ml syrup

The syrup is optional, to mask the bitter taste of morphine. Morphine can also be administered as an aqueous solution. This syrup can be inserted through a gastrostomic tube.

Previously, the so-called 'Brompton cocktail' was prescribed. It is a morphine solution containing cocaine and alcohol to avoid the initial drowsiness caused by morphine and preserve the solution longer. The Brompton syrup is better not used.

Cocaine can lead to hallucinations and suicide, while the initial drowsiness from morphine only lasts a few days. Alcohol is an irritant to an inflamed or dry mouth, which is a frequent consequence of chemotherapy or radiotherapy treatment in cancer patients.

Viable alternatives to syrup are the so-called slow-release pills such as MS Contin®. MS Contin® is available in tablets of 10, 30, 60 and 100 mg. They work for 12 hours and therefore must be taken twice a day, at 8 a.m. and 8 p.m. for example. MS Contin® should not be crushed in order to administer it via a gastrostomic probe, since this negates the 12-hour slow-release effect.

Two viable substitutes for oral morphine are hydromorphone (Palladone®) and oxycodone (Oxycontin®). Hydromorphone is more than 7 times as powerful as morphine, and oxycodone is 1.5 times stronger than morphine. The slow-release form of Palladone®, which also works for 12 hours, comes in tablets of 4, 8, 16 and 24 mg, with 4 mg being equivalent to 30 mg of MS Contin®. The short-acting preparation (4 hours) exists with 1.3 mg and 2.6 mg hydromorphone. It is similar to 10 and 20 mg morphine. Oxycontin® also works for 12 hours and is available in pill form of 5, 10, 20, 40 and 80 mg. Ten milligrams of Oxycontin® corresponds to about 15 mg MS Contin®. Oxynorm® is a short-acting (4 hours) melting tablet and is available in 5, 10 and 20 mg. It is also available for injection (10 mg/ml). Of all strong opioids (morphine mimetica) Oxycontin® – which also has a marked effect on neuropathic pain – is the most commonly used worldwide.

3. Starting with morphine

When starting with oral morphine, it is best to start with the short-acting preparations such as the syrup. If the patient has been through step 2 of the pain ladder a dosage of 10 mg of morphine can be given, but if the patient immediately starts on step 3 it is safer to start with 5 mg, particularly in elderly patients. The dose can be increased by roughly 50 per cent, for example 10 mg, then 15 mg, and then rounded to 20 mg etc.) every 4 hours until the patient is pain free. There is no maximum daily dose of morphine. The maximum is determined by the level of pain. Most patients, however, rarely exceed 200 mg of morphine per day. Above this dose the recommended increase in dosage is 30 per cent of the previous dose.

In this way most morphine-responsive pain can be controlled within 48 hours.

An alternative is to administer 20–60 mg in slow-release pill form, such as 2 × 10 or 30 mg of MS Contin® or 2 × 4 mg of Palladone or 2 × 20 mg of Oxycontin®. The dose is adjusted by increasing the amount by 50 per cent at a time. If 2 × 30 mg appears inadequate, the following day 2 × 45 mg (rounded down to 2 × 40 mg) is given: 1 × 10 and 1 × 30 mg twice daily. The frequency does not change: MS Contin® is not administered 3 or 4 times a day, because this leads to accumulation and permanent drowsiness and confusion.

4. When oral morphine is not possible

Sometimes the patient is unable to swallow the morphine. This happens if the patient has temporary swallowing problems, for example after radiation therapy for throat cancer, or is too weak, vomiting or unconscious. Sometimes the patient refuses to comply due to confusion or mental illness.

In such instances, the doctor must resort to parenteral administration: an intravenous or subcutaneous infusion, an epidural catheter via the rectum, or resorption through the skin via a patch.

The intravenous option is best avoided if possible because the patient loses their independence and is generally obliged to stay in hospital. The patient can carry a subcutaneous infusion bag – the so-called portable syringe driver (see p.125).

Morphine patches can also be used. The patch is stuck to the patient's skin and the morphine is released constantly and penetrates through the skin into the body.

Durogesic® patches contain fentanyl, a product developed for anaesthesia. It is about 150 times more powerful than morphine. The patches need to be replaced every 3 days. They are available with 12.5, 25, 50, 75 and 100 µg/hour release rates, approximately equivalent to 30, 60, 120, 180 and 240 mg of oral morphine a day respectively. These patches can be cut. When switching from oral morphine to Durogesic® it is important to remember that the patch is only effective after 12 hours and so should be put on at the same time as the last dose of MS Contin®.

Durogesic® is convenient to administer, but because it works for 72 hours, the patch cannot be used for the optimal daily dose of pain medication. Most patients still often take oral morphine as well, for example with breakthrough pain (see p.217). Durogesic® can be used to absorb most chronic pain. Oral morphine is added to absorb the daily fluctuations.

Similar patches with buprenorphine (Transtec®) are available, with release rates of 35, 52.5, 70 mg/hour (35 mg/hour corresponds to a daily dose of oral morphine of less than 120 mg). These patches can also be cut, and last 72 hours.

5. Some rules of thumb

The dose of morphine varies depending on whether it is administered orally, intravenously, subcutaneously, via a patch or via the rectum.

When changing from one form to another it is best to calculate the correct dosage of each based on the oral daily dose. This is definitely useful in patients who have a patch, intravenously administered morphine and occasionally some morphine syrup or Oxynorm®.

When switching from oral morphine to intravenous or subcutaneous morphine, the daily oral dose is divided by 3 and 2 respectively. If a daily dose of 60 mg (2 × 30 mg) of MS Contin® relieves the pain, then the equivalent via an intravenous drip will be 60 mg divided by 3, i.e. 20 mg of morphine every 24 hours. The parenteral dose will be lower because when morphine is taken orally approximately two-thirds is broken down by the liver. The indications for inserting an epidural catheter are limited. Moreover, a catheter is very cumbersome for home care.

Suppositories are not often used. This is probably explained by the regularity – 6 times a day – with which they should be inserted. Another possibility is MS Contin® via the rectum, whereby the absorption is shown to be equivalent to oral administration.

The syringe driver (subcutaneous pain pump)

In palliative care, a simple pain pump that runs on batteries is used regularly. A plastic disposable syringe is filled with soluble active products and then mounted on the pump, hence the name 'syringe driver' or 'injection actuator'. The medicine is administered continuously subcutaneously via a catheter and a (butterfly) needle, normally for a period of 24 hours. In addition to morphine (hence the name 'pain pump') the following products are usually administered:

- anti-emetics: haloperidol (Haldol®);
- anticholinergic agents: scopolamine;
- sedatives/anti-convulsants: midazolam (Dormicum®).

Other products are also administered using the syringe pump: alizapride (Litican®), dexamethasone (Aacidexam®), furosemide (Lasix®), hyoscine butylbromide (Buscopan®), levomepromazine (Nozinan®), methylprednisolone (Solu-Medrol®), metoclopramide (Primperan®), octreotide (Sandostatin®), promethazine (Phenergan®), ranitidine (Zantac®).

The following products are to be avoided because of incompatibility: chlorpromazine, NSAIDs, except nimesulide (Mesulid®), diazepam (Valium®).

6. Side-effects

Morphine has a crippling effect on the intestine and always causes constipation. For this reason a (preventive) laxative, such as Prunazine® syrup or Laxoberon® drops, must always be taken with it. The patient should be encouraged to drink a lot (fruit juice) and to eat fruit and high-fibre food. With terminal patients, the latter is rarely possible.

In most patients, nausea and vomiting is possible for the first few days. When this is expected – when the patient has experienced heavy vomiting during earlier chemotherapy, for example – then an anti-vomiting agent such as Litican® or Primperan® can be used. Haldol® (5–10 drops 3 times daily) is commonly used, and because haloperidol is a neuroleptic, frequently prescribed in psychiatry, the patient must be informed that it is being used.

In the beginning the patient may experience drowsiness, dizziness and confusion. Again it is important to inform patients of this possibility in advance so they know what to expect and don't panic or reject (often definitively) the medication.

Multifocal myoclonus or muscle twitches can occur with very high doses. If it is not possible to reduce the dose, an anti-convulsant such as clonazepam (Rivotril®)

can be given. A limited number of patients experience temporary urinary retention. A one-time probe is often sufficient. Itching, excessive sweating – especially at night – and a dry mouth are also potential side-effects.

Should one drive under the influence of morphine?

Empirical observations and recent studies show that driving is indeed possible when the patient is taking a stable daily dose, although obviously not during the initial phase or when the dose has been adjusted.

7. Morphine intolerance

In rare cases, patients are morphine intolerant. This may result in a paralysis of the digestive system, combined severe gastric stasis characterised by 'feeling full', anorexia, persistent vomiting and wind. A possible solution is to prescribe an anti-vomiting drug such as Primperan® or to switch to a different opioid such as hydromorphone (Palladone®), oxycodone (Oxycontin®) or methadone (Mephenon®). The patient may experience hallucinations – deceased family members walking past the bed or small rodents in the corners of the room – cognitive impairment and maladaptive behaviour (dysphoria). Haloperidol (Haldol®, 3–5 mg in the evening) may provide a solution; otherwise switch to an alternative opioid. Another uncommon symptom is generalised itching, due to the release of histamine in the skin. If taking an antihistamine such as Zyrtec® (1 per day, or Fenistil® 3 × 1 per day) doesn't help, try a different opioid.

8. Changing to a different opioid

Opioid rotation

Sometimes patients want to change from one opioid preparation to another because of unbearable side-effects and inadequate pain relief. Sometimes a change can improve major side-effects such as cognitive impairment, hallucinations, sedation, nausea and vomiting and even myoclonus. Problems are sometimes attributed to metabolites of morphine. Morphine is metabolised in the liver in the inactive morphine-3-glucuronide and active morphine-6-glucuronide (M6G). M6G is much more powerful than morphine itself. Normally these products are excreted by the kidneys. In some circumstances, such as kidney failure, they can accumulate in the body.

Morphine may in these circumstances be replaced by hydromorphone, oxycodone, fentanyl or methadone, which have no toxic degradation products.

Relative strength of analgesics (oral)

	strength relative to morphine	duration (hrs)
morphine	1	4
Aspirin®	$1/200$	4
tilidine (Valtran®)	$1/7$	4*
codeine	$1/10$	3–6

tramadol (Tradonal®, Contramal®, Dolzam®)	⅕	4–6*
fentanyl (Durogesic®) transdermal	100–150	
oxycodone	1.5	4
hydromorphone	7	4
methadone (Mephenon®)	5–10**	8–10

* Also exists in slow-release form, lasting 12 hours.

** A one-off administration of 5 mg methadone (Mephenon®) is approximately 7.5 mg of morphine. However, methadone remains in the blood for a long time and repeated administration causes an accumulation of methadone. This makes it 5–10 times stronger than expected (see section below on methadone).

With high doses of morphine (more than 2000 mg orally per day) the inactive metabolite morphine-3-glucuronide will partially neutralise the effect of the morphine. In such instances it is best to take between a half and a quarter of the calculated equivalent dose in opioid rotation.

Replacing morphine with methadone

Methadone is totally different to morphine. In addition to acting as an opioid, it interferes with the NMDA receptor and also has an effect on neuropathic pain. Methadone can also be prescribed to patients with severe kidney failure because, unlike morphine, its metabolism and excretion do not depend on the kidney.

Given that the maximum effect of methadone only kicks in after a few days, the dose must be carefully titrated and shouldn't be used in the patient's last days.

How to start with methadone

Patients with kidney failure, for example, who have not yet taken any morphine preparations can start with 5–10 mg methadone twice a day. If necessary they can add 5 mg every 3 hours. This dose is reviewed every 4–6 days.

For patients who are already taking morphine, the Morley and Makin model can be used.

Stopping morphine

- Start the methadone with a dose equivalent to one tenth of the daily dose of oral morphine, up to a maximum of 30 mg methadone.
- This dose can be taken every 3 hours according to need.
- On day 6 the daily dose of the last 2 days is taken into account and one can administer this in 2 doses (one every 12 hours). In addition a similar or even smaller dose can be taken every 3 hours if necessary.
- If this emergency dose still needs to be taken, the daily dose should be increased by a half or a third every 4–6 days.
- Usually patients do not require more than 40 mg of methadone per day.

9. The problem of breakthrough pain

Even with good pain control in place the patient might still experience flare-ups of severe pain at unpredictable moments (for example abdominal cramps) and/or at predictable moments (incidental pain), for example when treating a pressure wound. The emergency dose to combat breakthrough pain is, as a rule of thumb, one sixth (at high doses one tenth) of the daily morphine dose. A patient whose pain is kept under control with 2×100 mg MS Contin® (a daily dose of 200 mg) will need an emergency dose of one sixth of 200, or 30 mg of short-acting oral morphine. This equates to 30 mg morphine syrup or approximately 20 mg Oxynorm® pills. For an equivalent subcutaneous dose, the oral dose is divided in two and 15 mg of morphine is administered subcutaneously and not, as too often happens, half of a 10 mg morphine ampoule. Oral fentanyl was recently introduced as a lollipop (Actiq®) or as buccal pills: Effentora® of 100, 200, 400, 600 and 800 µg respectively.

10. Stopping with morphine: the problem of withdrawal

Stopping morphine 'cold turkey' results in withdrawal symptoms. This happens frequently after surgery, when medication is stopped beforehand and forgotten afterwards. The deprivation is the result of the physical dependence. The severity depends on the quantity and length of time the morphine has been used.

The withdrawal syndrome develops after 6–12 hours and manifests itself in anxiety, nervousness, irritability and feeling hot and cold alternately. The person concerned can be described as a 'wet patient': salivation, runny eyes, loss of nasal fluid, sneezing, sweating and goose bumps. These withdrawal symptoms peak after 1–3 days and may result in nausea and vomiting as well as stomach cramps, insomnia, anxiety, excitement and fear, even multifocal myoclonus.

Withdrawal symptoms can be explained as follows: the continuous administration of certain products results in the shutting down of various brain functions. The human body tries to compensate by extra activity. When a person suddenly stops taking the product, compensation mechanisms remain, even 'overshoot' and manifest as withdrawal symptoms.

So when the pain is suddenly controlled by a given intervention and the morphine is no longer needed, the patient should be gently weaned off the morphine. As a rule of thumb, to wean a patient off morphine derivatives, the daily dose should be decreased by 75 per cent each day.

11. How to treat an overdose

It rarely happens, but can occur due to an incorrect dosage or when a patient has attempted self-medication. Clinically, a morphine overdose manifests itself in respiratory depression, sedation and miosis. In these cases the morphine-antagonist naloxone, which primarily works on the respiratory depression, is used. At higher concentrations naloxone is also effective against deep sedation and raises the analgesic effect of morphine. It may even provoke deprivation. One should therefore not give too much. Intravenous naloxone is effective for 15–90 minutes, which is less than morphine. For respiratory depression 100–200 μg generally suffices. In emergencies 100 μg can be given intravenously using a venepuncture every 3 minutes until it achieves an acceptable result.

12. Morphine for unbearable pain

In some cases, the patient literally writhes in pain and should be treated quickly. Communication with the patient is often no longer possible.

When the patient is no longer being treated with morphine – or where it is not known whether they are being treated with morphine – start with an infusion of 0.5 mg of morphine per hour. This may be preceded by a subcutaneous injection of 5–10 mg of morphine.

When the patient is already taking morphine but neither the opioid nor the dosage is known, then 2–5 mg morphine should be administered through the vein every 10 minutes until the pain has been relieved. The daily intravenous dose is then calculated. If 4×2 mg was given in 40 minutes to obtain acceptable pain relief, then this corresponds to 12 mg per hour or 12 mg $\times$ 24, which is 288 mg per day.

Adjuvants

Painkillers can be used on all steps of the pain ladder in conjunction with the so-called adjunctive medication. The adjuvants either improve the effect of the painkillers (then also called co-analgesics) or reduce the side-effects, e.g. laxatives, anti-emetics and psychostimulants.

1. Co-analgesics
Antidepressants as co-analgesics

Antidepressants are used due to their beneficial effect on neuropathic pain and other chronic pain syndromes such as migraines, lower-back pain, cancer pain and fibromyalgia. Substances such as the tricyclic antidepressants – amitriptyline (Redomex®, Tryptizol®), imipramine (Tofranil®), clomipramine (Anafranil®) – also have, in addition to their antidepressant effect, an analgesic effect on neuropathic pain. Unlike antidepressants, whose effect manifests slowly after a few weeks, the effect on the pain can be felt after just one week. Start with an initial dose of 10–25 mg in the evening, and increase it by 25 mg every 3 days until reaching a final dose of 100–150 mg/day, to be taken in the evening. Some patients complain of a dry mouth or sleepiness.

More recently developed products such as Efexor® also work as analgesics. The starting dose is 37.5 mg per day, increasing to 75 mg, and exceptionally up to a maximum of 225 mg per day, taken at one time in slow-release form (Efexor XL®).

Anticonvulsants for neuropathic pain

Anticonvulsants can be used on their own, but can also be combined with antidepressants. An example of an anticonvulsant is carbamazepine (Tegretol®). The starting dose is 100 mg twice a day. In order to minimise the side-effects (double vision, movement disorders, dizziness), the dose is increased by 200 mg per week to a maximum of 600 mg. Valproate (Depakine®) and Depakine® Chrono (300 and 500 mg respectively) are interesting substances for relieving neuropathic pain, and should be taken in the evening. Taking Depakine® once a day can cause side-effects such as stomach pain, vomiting, drowsiness and vertigo. These are less pronounced when the optimal dose is built up gradually. Start with 500 mg Depakine Chrono® in the evening and increase the dose to 3×500 mg in a week. Fenytoine (Diphantoine®) can be administered in one go of 300 mg or 2×150 mg at an interval of several hours.

Pregabalin (Lyrica®) is another interesting product. Start with 2×75 mg per day and increase to possibly 2×300 mg per day.

Other possible anticonvulsants include gabapentin (Neurontin®), lamotrigine (Lamictal®), topiramate (Topamax®) and tiagabine (Gabitril®).

Other products with an effect on specific receptors are used in chronic pain syndromes such as the α2 agonists clonidine (Dixarit®) and tizanidine (Sirdalud®). Baclofen (Lioresal®), a GABA agonist, or dextromethorfan (Actifed®) and ketamine (Ketalar®), two NMDA-receptor antagonists, can also be tried for neuropathic pain. These can be used in conjunction with co-analgesics such as mexiletine or calcitonin.

Benzodiazepines such as diazepam (Valium®), lorazepam (Temesta®) and oxazepam (Seresta®) can be used to combat muscle spasms. A classic example is spastic back-muscles caused by vertebral metastases.

Corticoids as analgesics

Corticoids are the prototype of efficient co-analgesics. They have many other useful features in controlling cancer patients' symptoms (see below).

Corticosteroids

Corticosteroids are hormones that are produced from cholesterol by the adrenal glands. They play a role in the water balance and the metabolism of glucose and proteins. Cortisol and corticosterone are natural glucocorticoids. Given their beneficial inhibitory properties on inflammation and oedemas, synthetic preparations with much higher activity were developed. Methylprednisolone (Medrol®) is 5 times stronger than cortisol, and dexamethasone (Aacidexam®) is 25 times stronger.

Prolonged use can result in side-effects as a result of the catabolism of proteins: thin skin, poor wound healing, susceptibility to infections, muscle weakness or myopathy. The redistribution of fat results in a typical 'buffalo neck'. Salt and fluid retention creates a swollen face (moonface) and high blood pressure. It causes osteoporosis due to reduced bone formation and increased bone resorption.

When treating incurable patients, corticosteroids are used primarily for their effect on inflammation and oedema (pain), the appetite, a feeling of wellbeing, breathing and vomiting. They have also been successfully used in some emergencies such as threatening cross lesions of the spinal cord, superior vena cava syndrome and brain metastases (see emergencies, p. 230).

The side-effects mentioned above are not so much of a concern with these patients as they usually only occur after a long time.

They are especially useful in managing nerve pain caused by compression of the nerve, for increased pressure inside the skull due to cerebral oedema caused by cerebral metastases and for bone cancer caused by metastases. Oedema from liver metastasis causes painful pressure on the liver and vomiting. Both symptoms can be treated with corticosteroids. Inflammatory oedema from a pronounced throat cancer is another example. Diffuse intestinal damage, as with ovarian cancer, also leads to oedema formation. The result is often a pronounced bowel obstruction with painful colic. Oedemas that block the gut cavity frequently respond spectacularly to corticosteroids, sometimes within months.

Methylprednisolone (Medrol®) is best administered in 2 doses. Corticosteroids can sometimes excite the patient, resulting in insomnia. This is prevented by giving the first dose in the morning, the second in the afternoon, and nothing in the evening.

When starting with corticosteroids, use a punch dose such as 32 mg Medrol® in the morning and in the afternoon. A striking improvement is often visible within 48 hours. Thereafter, the daily dose can be reduced to minimise the side-effects such as fluid retention, swollen face, pain and weakness in the legs. These side-effects are, however, not a reason to avoid using corticosteroids. In terms of life expectancy, the numerous benefits of these products are weighed against the long-term side-effects.

Bisphosphonates for bone pain

Bone tissue is a living organ that is constantly rebuilt. There are two different cell types: osteoblasts that promote bone formation and the osteoclasts which do the opposite. In normal circumstances there is a dynamic equilibrium between the two bone cells. In exceptional circumstances, such as after a leg fracture, the bone-forming cells are active. With bone metastases or osteoporosis, bone tissue is often destroyed.

Bisphosphonates are inorganic pyrophosphate analogues that have a blocking effect on osteoclasts, thereby decreasing bone resorption. They were originally developed to reduce hypercalcaemia, which can result from massive bone-marrow tumours. However, it soon became clear that bisphosphonates also have an analgesic effect on bone pain caused by metastases. Moreover, these substances can inhibit the development of new bone metastases. It has been shown that women with breast cancer exhibit less bone marrow cancer and suffer less from hypercalcaemia when treated regularly with bisphosphonates.

It's best to use the recently developed bisphosphonates such as zoledronic acid (Zometa®), alendronate (Fosamax®), ibandronic acid (Bondronat®) and denosumab (Xgeva®). These products are often administered intravenously on a weekly basis followed by a monthly maintenance dose. They can also be taken orally or subcutaneously.

Radiopharmaceuticals for bone pain

Certain radioactive substances have a beneficial effect on bone pain caused by bone metastases. Products such as Strontium-89 are attracted by active bone remodelling to the place of the bone metastasis because they are structurally very similar to calcium. The use of these products is limited, however, because of potential bone-marrow damage, with anaemia as a result. In addition, it is a very expensive treatment.

2. Adjuvants to counter the side-effects of painkillers

Laxatives should always be administered as a preventive measure, and anti-vomiting pills can be helpful, especially when starting or increasing the morphine dose (see p. 224).

Psychostimulating substances, or psychostimulants

Methylphenidate (Rilatin®) is a short-acting amphetamine. It is used for lethargic narcolepsy patients and hyperkinetic children with ADHD (Attention Deficit Hyperactivity Disorder). Methylphenidate is given to cancer patients taking high doses of painkillers to combat drowsiness, to improve cognitive functions and to lighten the depressed mood and reduce fatigue. The product also exhibits analgesic properties. The starting dose is 2.5–5 mg in the morning and afternoon and is increased by 5–10 mg per week until it has an acceptable effect. The daily dose usually does not exceed 60 mg (divided into 2 doses). Methylphenidate may, however, lead to anorexia, weight loss and insomnia, which certainly is not desired in cancer patients. Opioid-induced sleepiness is also counteracted by modafinil (Provigil®), which is also administered to multiple sclerosis sufferers to combat fatigue. However, this product is quite expensive.

Cannabinoids

The most active constituent of cannabis is tetrahydrocannabinol (THC). There is a lot of controversy around the added value of cannabinoids. Since the massive use of marijuana by hippies in the seventies it has had many properties attributed to it. Apart from obvious effects on the central nervous system such as hallucinations, it also stimulates the appetite and has anti-vomiting as well as euphoriant and relaxing, even analgesic, effects. Ten milligrams of THC has an equivalent analgesic effect to 60 mg codeine. The problem remains the very limited therapeutic margin: this is the margin between a dose with a beneficial effect, such as pain relief, and an unwanted side-effect such as hallucinations.

Medication-based support for anxiety

Anticipatory anxiety before an examination is best treated (medically) with short-acting benzodiazepines such as midazolam (Dormicum®), alprazolam (Xanax®) or lorazepam (Temesta®).

Longer-acting products such as clonazepam (Rivotril®), prazepam (Lysanxia®) and diazepam (Valium®) can be used for long-term anxiety prevention.

Neuroleptics such as haloperidol (Haldol®) (less sedative) or thioridazine (Melleril®) (sedative) can be useful, respectively, for anxious but also confused patients, or medically induced akathisia.

Certain antidepressants also counter anxiety and reduce panic attacks, for example citalopram (Cipramil®) and paroxetine (Seroxat®).

Medication-based support for anorexia-cachexia syndrome

Effective medications include metoclopramide, progestins, and corticosteroids. Products with a potential value include thalidomide, anabolic steroids, cannabinoids, melatonin, growth hormones, omega-3 fatty acids and NSAIDs. Useless resources include cyproheptadine and hydrazine sulphate.

Products without value (worthless products)

Cyproheptadine (Periactin®) is an antihistamine used for children with allergies which also causes weight gain. In practice, it is of very little value.

Hydrazine sulphate prevents the conversion of proteins into glucose in rats. It also inhibits TNF (tumour necrosis factor). In humans it has no effect.

Products whose effects are still under examination

Thalidomide is a fear-reducing sleeping medication with anti-vomiting properties. It was taken off the market 50 years ago after the disastrous experience with the deformed Softenon® babies born to women who had taken the drug during pregnancy. Recently it was discovered that this substance also interferes with the immune system, including inhibiting TNF. With AIDS patients it exhibits a positive impact on appetite, sense of wellbeing, nausea and insomnia. Patients also exhibited a noticeable weight gain after 8 weeks of treatment with 100–200 mg of thalidomide per day.

Male anabolic steroids such as nandrolone and oxandrolone have been used by bodybuilders for years because of the effect on their muscular development. These substances also have a positive influence on the weight of AIDS patients.

Although marijuana stimulates the appetite it does not result in increased body weight. The therapeutic area is very limited. And with cachectic patients, certain social circles struggle to accept the effects on the central nervous system, such as hallucinations. A trial treatment can be tried with the active ingredient of cannabis, dronabinol, 2.5 mg 2–3 times a day.

Melatonin can reduce the TNF levels in advanced cancer patients. It can not only impact on body weight but also the fatigue in patients undergoing chemotherapy.

Growth hormones promote protein production and their influence on the insulin-like growth factor-1 (IGF-1) causes the muscle cells to develop.

Omega-3 fatty acids such as eicosapentanoic acid (EPA) are unsaturated fats that are found in fish oil. They have an effect on the immune system and reduce the concentration of various cytokines and proteolysis-inducing factors (PIF). In cancer patients with cachexia there is also an effect on the weight.

NSAIDs reduce Interleukin-6, and meloxicam (Mobic®) reduces the growth of tumours in mice.

Products that have proved their worth

Metoclopramide (Primperan®) is useful in treating chronic nausea. It also promotes gastric emptying.

Progestins such as megestrol (Megace®) or medroxyprogesterone acetate (Provera®) appear to be a second alternative. They result in weight gain in hormone-sensitive cancer cases when used for hormone therapy. They stimulate the appetite and have a positive impact on nausea, pain, energy levels, general comfort and body weight. The effect is only noticeable from 6 weeks after daily administration of up to 800 mg per day. The patient should be informed of this long latency. They also appear to have a longer-lasting effect than corticosteroids. In addition, they appear to have an inhibiting effect on TNF. Provera® is available as syrup (2 × 5ml per day), which is very useful for patients who are already overwhelmed with swallowing all kinds of pills.

Corticosteroids such as Medrol® (2 × 16 mg per day) stimulate the appetite and reduce nausea and vomiting. They are euphoriants and have a positive effect on asthenia and general comfort. Their mode of action mechanism is not clear. Unfortunately, the effect is rather short lived: 3–4 weeks. It is therefore best to keep them till the final stage or to use them for short periods.

Medication for dyspnea

Opioids

Subjective difficulty in breathing can be clearly highlighted with morphine preparations. Dyspnea improves by reducing the speed of breathing. A first test dose of 5 mg of morphine should be given either by mouth (for example morphine syrup) or subcutaneously. This can then be repeated every 4 hours. If this is moderately successful, the dose can be adjusted to 10 mg every 4 hours. It is also possible to switch to slow-release oral morphine or a subcutaneous or intravenous drip. With patients who are already on morphine, the daily dose should be increased by 50 per cent.

Other possibilities

The role of mucolytics such as Lysomucil® to loosen phlegm in order to help the patient's breathing is dubious. They are better omitted in seriously ill patients who are usually already exposed to numerous drugs. If the direct cause of the dyspnea is not immediately clear, it is possible to trial therapy with corticosteroids. Anxiety-reducing benzodiazepines such as Xanax® or Temesta® often help.

There is no risk of respiratory depression with either opioids or benzo-diazepines.

Prevention and treatment of constipation: possible laxatives
Fibre-rich products such as psyllium husks cause fluid absorption in the intestine, resulting in a voluminous bowel movement. They are therefore rarely used in palliative care.

Osmotic products also attract moisture to and ensure a moist, smooth bowel movement:
- salt solutions such as Movicol® bags 3×1 per day, or more drastically Colopeg®, Transipeg® or Prepacol®, which are also used for bowel cleansing before a bowel examination;
- sugar solutions that do not pass through the stomach and so remain in the intestine, such as:
  - lactulose: Duphalac® or Bifiteral® bags, 3×1 per day;
  - sorbitol: bags, 3×1 per day.

Contact laxatives stimulate the intestinal tract, thereby promoting bowel movements and the passing of stools. They can also cause intestinal cramps, diarrhoea and even hypokalaemia. Examples are:
- Laxoberon® drops, 3×10 drops per day;
- Senokot®, 3×1 per day;
- Dulcolax®, 2–3 per day.

Softeners help to soften the stool and facilitate its passing. Examples are:
- paraffin oil, 1–2 tablespoons per day;
- DulcoEase®.

There are also enemas that are inserted via the rectum. Examples are:
- Fleet®;
- Microlax®.

Glycerine suppositories – less aggressive on the intestinal lining – may also be prescribed.

For patients with serious faecal impaction, it is worth trying Movicol®, 8 bags per day (2 per hour) or Colopeg®. Another possibility is carefully to insert a rectal probe above the impacted stool and spray it with glycerine. An application with Lysomucil® (10 ampoules to 1 litre of lukewarm water) can also be tried.

If all these attempts fail, the only remaining possibility is the manual removal of the stool. The patient should be sedated 30 minutes beforehand with a subcutaneous injection of 5 mg of Dormicum®. This clearly illustrates the expression 'prevention is better than cure'.

A new product for adults is methylnaltrexonbromide (Relistor®). It is the first in a new class of peripheral μ-opioid receptor antagonists which reverses the obstipation effects of opioids in the gastro-intestinal tract without compromising the pain treatment. Twelve milligrams of Relistor® should be administered subcutaneously every 2 days. If the constipation persists, this can be preceded by 12 mg per day for 3 days. Injections should only be given near a toilet, because the effect can be very quick (within 30 minutes). Classic laxatives should not, however, be stopped.

Medication for delirium
Agitation/hallucinations: 2 mg haloperidol (Haldol®) orally or subcutaneously every 6 hours. For extreme agitation it is often desirable to administer Haldol® more frequently: 2 mg intravenously or subcutaneously every 15–30 minutes for the first hour and then 2 mg every hour. Olanzapine (Zyprexa®), 2.5–10 mg per day, can also be used. It is important to bring this situation under control as soon as possible, not only for the patient but also for the family. Sometimes sedatives can be used, such as chlorpromazine or even midazolam (Dormicum®): 1 mg per hour until there is a clinical response. The problem with benzodiazepines, however, is that when administered without adding Haldol®, they only act as sedatives, without any effect on cognitive functions. This may exacerbate the confusion and/or anxiety.

Terminal turmoil/agitation: delirium during the dying days
Possible medication is:
- midazolam (Dormicum®), up to 10 mg administered subcutaneously every 2 hours, or 60 mg per day (subcutaneously) and titration (syringe driver);
- clonazepam (Rivotril®), 0.5 mg orally or subcutaneously every 12 hours, or 2 mg daily subcutaneously and titration;
- diazepam (Valium®), up to 10–20 mg rectally or intravenously every 6 hours and titration;
- Lorazepam (Temesta®), up to 2.5 mg orally every 2–4 hours and titration.
If benzodiazepines do not help then try:
- phenobarbital, 100–200 mg subcutaneously every 4–6 hours and titration.

The role of antidepressants for patients with life-threatening conditions
Although the optimal use of antidepressants in cancer patients is not clear, various observations suggest that they may be useful in some patients. It is best to choose an antidepressant whose side-effects reflect the patient's situation. A patient with delayed psychomotor reactions will derive more benefit from a more activating antidepressant such as methylphenidate (Rilatin®) or fluoxetine (Prozac®). If the depressed patient is also agitated it may be best to prescribe a more sedating antidepressant such as nortryptiline (Allegron®) or mirtazapine (Remergon®). Other useful products are Trazolan® (100 mg and 150 mg slow release), Cipramil® (20 mg), Seroxat® or Paxil® (20 mg) and Serlain® (50 mg).

Antiemetics (anti-vomiting)
The same receptors are often found on different levels (see p. 113), such as receptors for 5 hydroxytryptamine, serotonin, dopamine, acetylcholine, or histamine. This explains why the same product is effective for different causes of vomiting.

The central nervous system: 'central vomiting'
- anticholinergic agents: scopolamine ampoules with 0.25 mg; subcutaneously every 4 hours;
- corticosteroids for cerebral oedema from brain tumours or metastases (Medrol®, Aacidexam®, 5 mg ampoules subcutaneously or orally);
- anxiolytics for anxiety (Xanax®).

The chemoreceptor trigger zone
- Dopamine 2 antagonists: haloperidol (Haldol®), chlorpromazine, metoclopramide (Primperan®), domperidone (Motilium®), olanzapine (Zyprexa®), as well as amitriptyline (Redomex®) and promethazine (Phenergan®);
- 5HT3 antagonists such as ondansetron (Zofran®).

The vomiting centre (area postrema)
- Serotonin antagonists: amitryptiline (Redomex®);
- antihistamines: promethazine (Phenergan®), chlorpromazine;
- anticholinergics: scopolamine, hyoscine butylbromide (Buscopan®), promethazine (Phenergan®), chlorpromazine.

Peripheral nerves
- Gastrokinetic agents:
  - metoclopramide (primperan®), domperidone (Motilium®), ondansetron (Zofran®).

Irritation
- Maalox®, Mylanta®, Gaviscon®;
- H2 antihistamines: Zantac®, Tagamet®;
- proton-pump inhibitors: Dakar®, Logastric®, Losec®, Nexiam®, Pantozol®, Pariet®.

Obstruction
- Haloperidol (Haldol®), hyoscine hydrobromide (scopolamine), hyoscine butylbromide (Buscopan®).

The anticholinergics hyoscine butylbromide (Buscopan®) and hyoscine hydrobromide (scopolamine) are structurally related and have a similar action. The only difference is that scopolamine penetrates the brain, while Buscopan® does not. For this reason only scopolamine is effective against central vomiting, but high doses can cause confusion. Both are effective when death rattle sounds.

Treating ascites

Ascites puncture

An imaginary line is drawn between the navel and the left crista iliaca (spina iliaca anterior superior) and a mark is made two-thirds away from the navel. The right side is avoided because there is a risk of pricking an enlarged liver. An intramuscular Terumo needle can be used to evacuate bright green liquid moisture. If the ascites fluid is more dense and high in protein, it is better to use a 2mm-thick Venflon or Pleurocath needle, whereby the plastic cannula is inserted in the abdominal cavity. For the latter option, a local anesthetic should be used, for example spraying ethyl chloride on the skin or injecting 5–10ml of lidocaine (Xylocaïne®) up the peritoneum.

The connecting line of an infusion bag is fitted on the needle with the cut off end hanging down in a collection system such as a bucket. One can also use vacuum bottles. Sterile gloves are not needed to perform these operations. There is little risk of bowel perforation, since the intestines themselves recede when the peritoneum is pierced. The frequency of ascites punctures in the palliative phase depends on the extent of the patient's suffering. The proteins lost in the puncture fluid are seldom restored in these patients. If the family doctor has insufficient experience to perform this operation, the patient can be referred to a day centre for these punctures.

Diuretics

A trial treatment with a diuretic such as spironolactone (Aldactone®) or furosemide (Lasix®) could be considered.

Aldactone® should be administered, 3×50mg per day, increased by 50mg per day until a daily dose of 400mg is reached. It can be combined with Lasix®, a maximum of 240mg per day.

Bladder irritation

Treatment should again be specific to the cause: antibiotics for infection, bladder catheter for urinary retention. As painkillers, NSAIDs can be used as well as products to prevent bladder spasms: flavoxate (Urispas®), 3×200mg per day, or oxybutynin (Ditropan®), 3×5mg, or tolterodine (Detrusitol®), 2×2mg per day.

Anti-diarrhoea agents

Anti-diarrhoea agents such as loperamide (Imodium®) may offer temporary relief: 1 pill after every loose stool up to 8 times a day.

Intestinal secretions can be absorbed by activated charcoal (Norit®) or products such as Actapulgite®, 3×1 sachet per day.

For persistent cases, codeine or morphine can be considered, or even Sandostatin® (see bowel obstruction).

Medication for bowel obstruction

The vomiting and discharge can be treated with Haldol®, Buscopan® or Sandostatin® and the colic pain with morphine. Laxatives must be stopped. In some cases, such as oedematous swelling of the intestines from micrometastases, test treatment with corticosteroids such as Medrol® or salt enemas can be tried. The bowel obstruction can often be kept under control with medication for some time.

The use of octreotide

Octreotide is a synthetic drug that mimics the somastatin hormone which, among other things, is responsible for the hormonal and neuroendocrine activity of the gastrointestinal tract. These are abnormally present in so-called NE-GEP (neuroendocrine gastroenteropancreatic) tumours. This can be used to treat persistent diarrhoea caused by these cancers, short bowel syndrome, graft-versus-host disease and after chemotherapy. It is a fairly expensive treatment and is therefore best used when all other options have been exhausted.

It can also be used to reduce gastrointestinal discharge from a bowel obstruction with extensive vomiting.

Octreotide (Sandostatin®) is administered via subcutaneous injections, 3×50–100 mg per day, and can be increased to 600 mg and exceptionally 1500 mg daily.

Treating hiccups

There are many different ways to try and stimulate the facial nervus phrenicus or the pharynx:
- drinking upside down from a glass;
- stimulation by alcohol or acid: liquor, vinegar or lemon juice;
- swallowing 2 teaspoons of sugar;
- pulling on your tongue;
- holding your breath and stretching your neck backwards;
- Valsalva-manoeuvre: pressing with closed throat;
- exercise pressure (manually) on the nose.

A distended stomach can be reduced by metoclopramide (Primperan®), 10–$20\,mg \times 3$ per day, domperidone (Motilium®), and by drinking peppermint water to relax the sphincter muscle of the oesophagus. It may be possible to release the air using a gastric tube.

A muscle relaxant can also be helpful, such as baclofen (Lioresal®), 2×10 mg per day, or nifedipine (Adalat®), 2×5 mg a day, if necessary increased to a maximum of 80 mg per day.

Reflexes in the central nervous system can be reduced by:
- chlorpromazine chlorohydrate 10–25 mg (magistral), 1 per day, increased as necessary but with care, as it has a strong sedative effect;
- haloperidol (Haldol®) in solution (10 drops equals 1 mg): 3–4 drops 10 times per day.

Benzodiazepines such as Temesta® or Valium® should definitely not be prescribed, as these can strengthen the hiccup.

Treatment of a persistent cough
Products that theoretically cure coughs such as Lysomucil® or Mucomyst® seem to have little effect in these cases.

For a persistent dry cough, it is best to prescribe the next level of treatment in addition to the treatment described above:

- Codeine, 6×10–60 mg per day; also available in syrup form: Bronchosedal®, 15 ml 3–6 times (equivalent to 13.5 mg codeine) per day;
- MS Contin®, 2×10–20 mg per day;
- Thebacone (Acedicon®), 3×5 mg per day.

Medication for itchiness
Several causes of itching such as cholestasis, can be treated with serotonin antagonists:

- paroxetine (Seroxat® or Aropax®), 20 mg per day;
- ondansetron (Zofran®), 2×8 mg per day and granisetron (Kytril®), 2×1 mg per day.

Other alternatives are:

- chlorpromazine, 3×25 mg per day;
- corticosteroids: dexamethasone, 1.5 mg per day;
- NSAIDs: naproxen (Naprosyn®), 3×250 mg per day;
- cimetidine (Tagamet®), 3×200–400 mg per day;
- even Redomex® and Haldol® at times.

Pleural puncture
After determining where the fluid has accumulated (dull percussion), the puncture point must be disinfected with Iso-Betadine or HAC (hospital antiseptic concentrate). The index finger is placed on and parallel to the 'bottom' rib under the puncture point and the ring finger on and parallel to the 'uppermost' rib. The middle finger then automatically falls in the intercostal region where the puncture should be made. A green Terumo-needle or pleural catheter is used to make the puncture towards the upper side in order to avoid the intercostal nerve. Ethyl chloride spray or a local anaesthetic, such as lidocaine hydrochloride (Xylocaïne®), can be used to numb the area, although it can usually be performed equally well without an anaesthetic since this also requires a prick. When the syringe fills, it means that it is in the pleural effusion between the lung membranes. The needle can then be connected to a pipe attached to a vacuum bottle, or if one is not available, if necessary the cut off end of a connecting line of an infusion bag can be hung in a container such as a bucket. When the patient starts to cough, it means that the needle point is in contact with the inner pleural membrane,

which means that most of the fluid has been drained. The needle is then carefully pulled out.

Emergencies

Spinal cord compression, brain metastases and superior vena cava syndrome may be treated with high doses of corticosteroids, for example methylprednisolone (Solu-medrol®, 80–250 mg per day intravenously, or Medrol®, 2 × 32 mg orally).

Excessive bleeding

Midazolam (Dormicum®) is used to put the patient to sleep quickly: 15–30 mg Dormicum® administered subcutaneously, depending on whether the patient is already taking benzodiazepines such as Valium® or Temesta®.

Morphine is used for the pain (ampoules of 30 mg per millilitre).

Products to treat the death rattle

Products that reduce the production of mucous such as the anticholinergics scopolamine, Buscopan® and Robinul®: 0.25 mg of scopolamine administered subcutaneously 4–6 times a day.

The technique of palliative sedation

Palliative sedation is used for patients suffering from untreatable forms of dyspnea, pain, nausea and vomiting, anxiety and delirium. The extent of sedation in principle happens after consultation with the patient or their family.

The best way is via a subcutaneous pain pump starting with an initial dose of 5–10 mg of Dormicum®. This is usually sufficient. Thereafter 60 mg are administered every 24 hours using a syringe driver. In some cases, 5–10 mg Dormicum® is not enough. In this situation the dose is doubled every 4 hours until the patient is sufficiently sedated (or half of the previous full dose is given every half hour). Usually one should not exceed 120 mg Dormicum® per 24 hours, although in extreme cases doses of 1000–1500 mg and even more can be used. An alternative to Dormicum® is levomepromazine (Nozinan®), 50–100 mg every 24 hours. Sedation can also be induced using diazepam (Valium®) suppositories or ampoules, 10 mg every hour until the patient is sufficiently sedated. Usually a maximum of 60 mg Valium® every 24 hours is enough.

If a patient has easy intravenous access, Dormicum® or Nozinan® can be administered through a vein, starting with half the subcutaneous dose. The bolus injection is administered slowly to avoid respiratory arrest. In difficult situations, when the patient struggles to be sedated, heavy sedatives such as the barbiturate thiopental can be used. This, incidentally, is the same drug used when performing euthanasia (except this time with an overdose). This adds to the confusion between palliative sedation and euthanasia (see below).

The technique of euthanasia

The first step is to insert a maintenance drip through a vein or portacath. In this way the technical aspects will not interfere at the time of application and all attention can be focussed on the patient and their relatives. The intravenous tubing allows the doctor, literally and figuratively, to remain discreetly in the background and make room for the other people present. The euthanasia can be performed by a quick injection (in 30–60 seconds) of an overdose of barbiturates (at least 2 g of thiopental) into the drip. The patient falls asleep immediately, quickly becomes comatose, and dies painlessly and calmly within 5 minutes. A third gram of thiopental is kept in reserve as a back-up. Some doctors first administer a soporific agent such as midazolam (Dormicum®) before injecting the barbiturates. Others later add a muscle-relaxant such as Mivacron® to be sure that the respiratory muscles remain paralysed. Experience has shown that an overdose of barbiturates administered rapidly is sufficiently effective. Some doctors let the patient drink a cocktail based on barbiturates (9 grams of natrium pentobarbital in water) preceded by an anti-vomiting drug and reassure the patient that they are nearby to administer more drugs (thiopental or Mivacron®) if it appears likely that the patient is going to come out of their barbiturate coma. In other words, the doctor carries the medical responsibility. However, it is very rare (less than 1 per cent of cases) that the patient will drink a lethal cocktail. Most patients are not capable (too weak, swallowing problems, vomiting) to do it themselves. A law that allows *only* this procedure, such as the proposed bill in the UK, is in fact discriminatory.

Euthanasia cocktail: mixture nontherapeutica pentobarbitali
　　sodium pentobarbital 9 g
　　alcohol 96° 16.2 g
　　aqua purificata 15 g
　　propylene glycol 10.4g
　　sodium saccharinate 250 mg
　　single syrup 65 g
　　aniseed essential oil 1 drop

In Belgium, because the Euthanasia Law does not specify how the euthanasia must be performed, the last procedure mentioned above is considered to be euthanasia and not 'assisted suicide'. A procedure can only be described as assisted suicide when the doctor gives or prescribes a lethal substance and the patient takes it *when the doctor is no longer present.*

The legislation applicable to assisted suicide in Belgium, however, is unclear. On the one hand, suicide is not a punishable offence in Belgium, so neither is helping a non-punishable act. On the other hand, the law can consider someone who commits suicide as a person in need. Failing to offer help to such a person can be interpreted as 'guilt by omission'. The fate of a doctor accused of assisting a suicide (prescribing or giving a lethal drug), depends on the judge's interpretation and attitude: help with a non-punishable act or guilty by omission. As a result, very few doctors tend to assist suicide.

Incidentally, morphine is certainly not the ideal euthanasia agent. It is a painkiller with drowsiness as an initial side-effect followed by respiratory depression in the event of an overdose. Mega-doses are required to make patients already taking morphine unconscious, let alone deeply comatose. In addition, the daily dose needs to be increased to maintain the coma, and often the patient can be comatose but alive for days. This is also true for patients who have never received morphine treatment.

Index